FRIENDSHIP
The Art of the Practice

Laurie Ellis-Young & Nancy Chakrin

TRISTAN PUBLISHING
Minneapolis

This book is dedicated to every woman we've ever called friend
beginning with our wonderful mothers: Leona (Jan) and Dorothy.

Laurie & Nancy

Copyright © 2010, Laurie Ellis-Young and Nancy Chakrin

Page 11: Claes Oldenburg and Coosje van Bruggen Spoonbridge and Cherry
1985-1988, Collection Walker Art Center, Minneapolis. Gift of Frederick R. Weisman in honor of his parents William and Mary Weisman, 1988 © Claes Oldenburg and Coosje van Bruggen
Page 33: "The Invitation" by Oriah from her book of the same name. Copyright © 1999. Published by HarperONE, San Fransisco. All rights reserved. Printed with the permission of the author. www.oriah.org.

Library of Congress Cataloging-in-Publication Data
Friendship : the art of the practice / [compiled] by Laurie Ellis-Young and Nancy Chakrin.
p. cm.
ISBN 978-0-931674-80-8 (alk. paper)
1. Female friendship--Pictorial works. 2. Yoga--Pictorial works. I. Ellis-Young, Laurie. II. Chakrin, Nancy.
HQ1233.F75 2010
302.3'4082--dc22
2010019731

TRISTAN PUBLISHING, INC.
2355 Louisiana Avenue North
Golden Valley, MN 55427

First Printir
Printed in Chin
Please visit www.tristanpublishing.co

INTRODUCTION

From the beginning this book seemed to have a life of its own, taking the authors along for a ride they never expected and connecting them with friends and yoginis ages 10-100.

A camera lens and yoga poses became vehicles for depicting and deepening connections with nature while honoring relationships - old and new, showing how both Friendship and Yoga transcend age, gender, race, religion and language.

"Friend beyond earthly constraints,
you come to me in my dreams where
we play and laugh like always;
I awaken rejuvenated by Love that
transcends all."

- Barbara Ann Caldwell

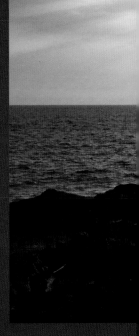

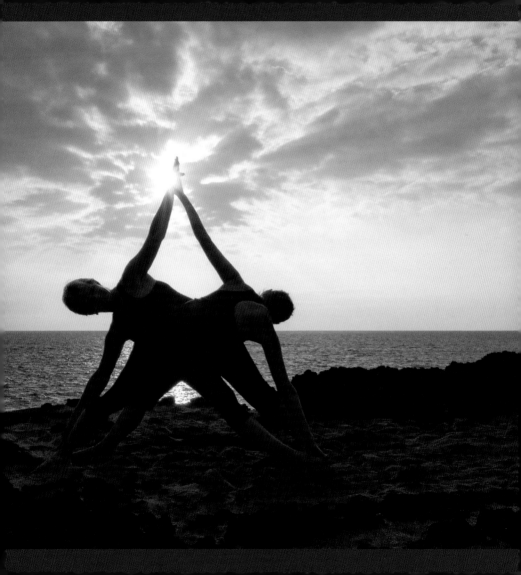

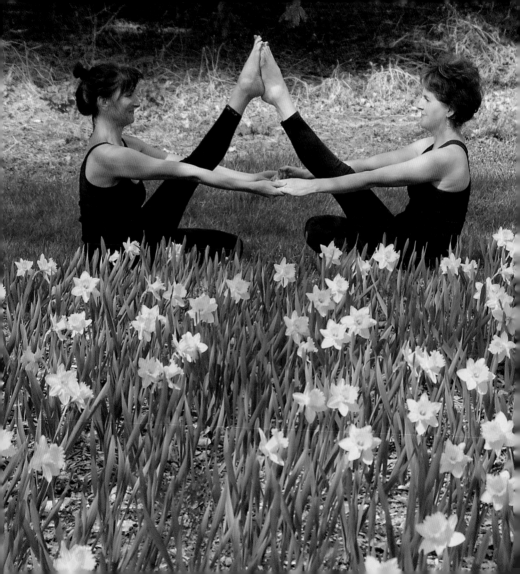

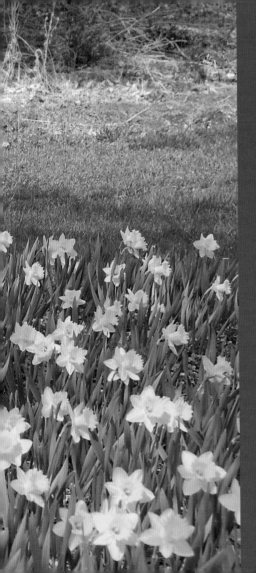

"If friends

were flowers,

I'd pick you."

- Unknown

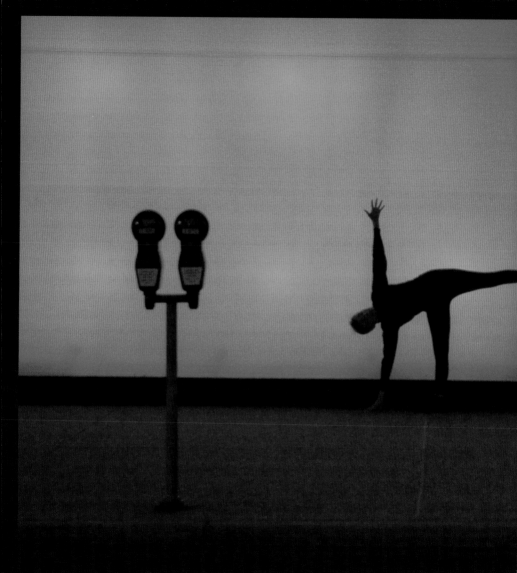

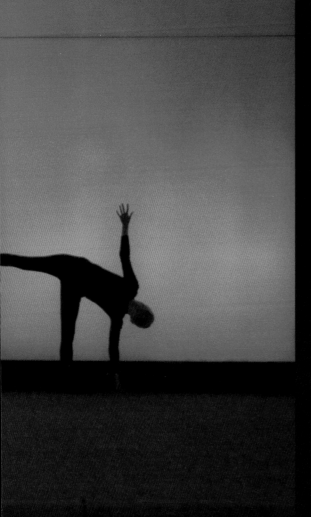

"True friendship

never expires."

- Neena Cohen

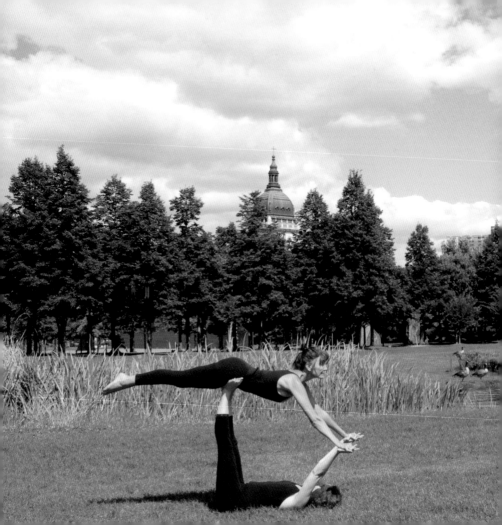

"I believe that friends are quiet angels who sit on our shoulders
and lift our wings when we forget how to fly."

- Unknown

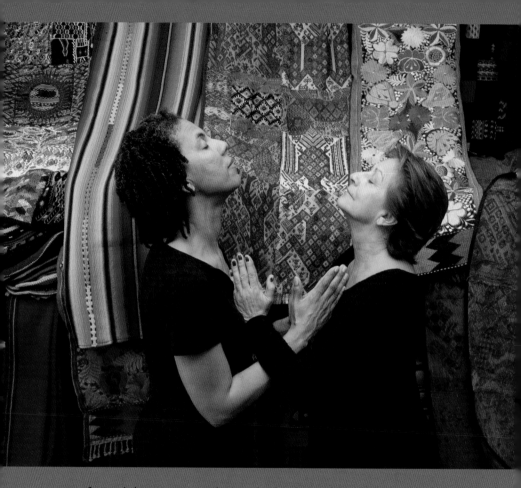

"True friendship is seen through the heart, not through the eyes."

- Unknown

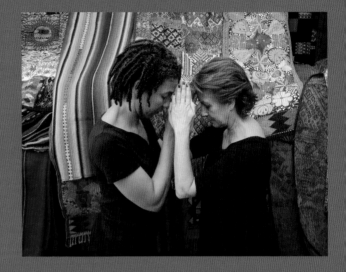

"I love you not only for what you are, but for what I am when I am with you."

- Unknown

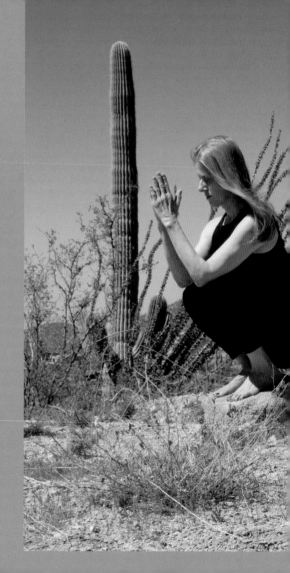

"A friend is someone
with whom silence is
as comfortable as
conversation."

- Joy Hayenga

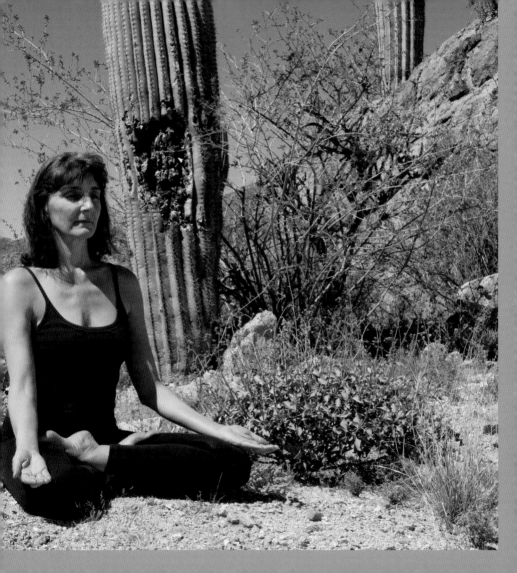

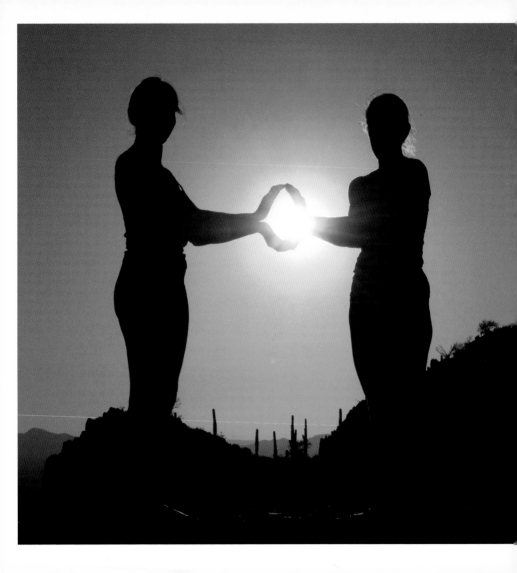

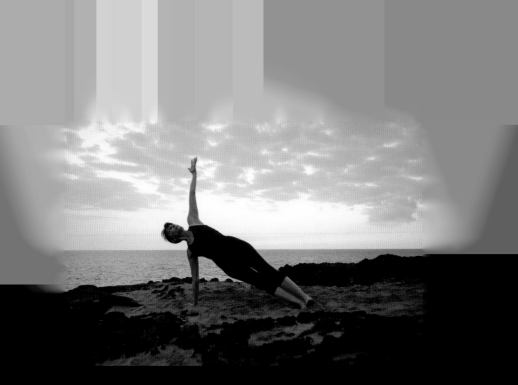

'The mind is either dwelling in the past or worrying about the future. But the body is always in the present moment. If you can bring your mind where

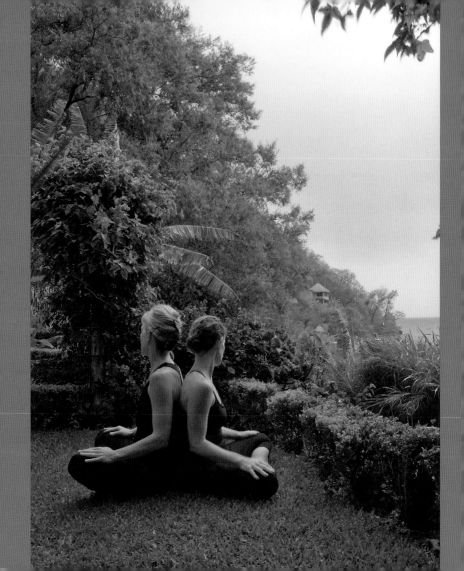

"Sometimes in friendships
you just need to look
the other way."

- L.E.Y.

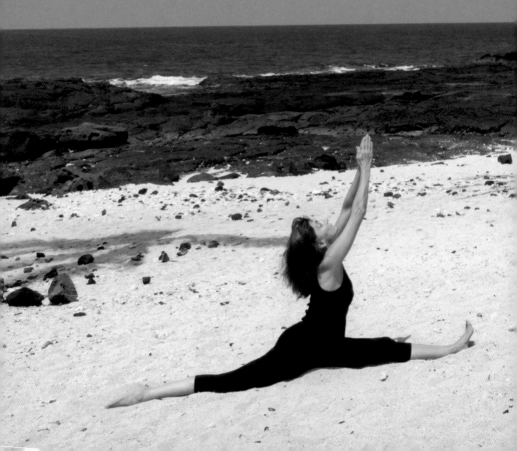

"My friend, silent amidst the sounds of the wind and waves, you exude a sense of peace. I love you for teaching me how to BE."

– Nancita

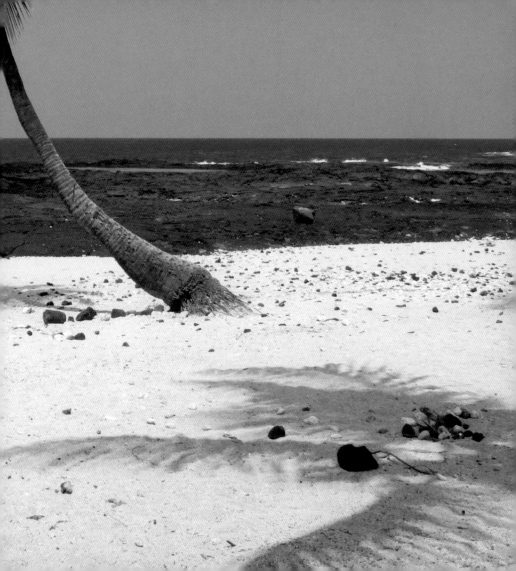

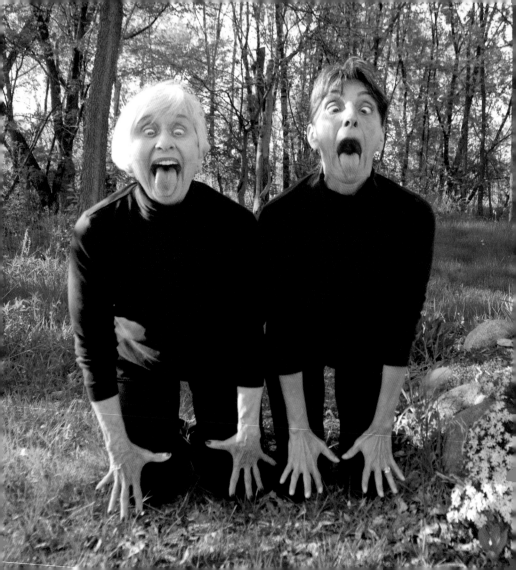

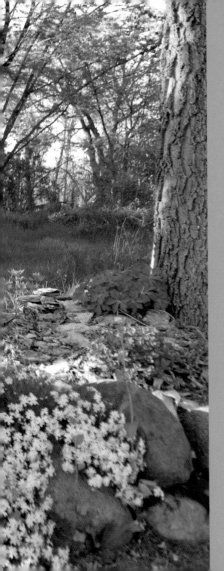

"How special the friend who will comfort me, challenge me, accept me and be crazy with me."

– L.E.Y

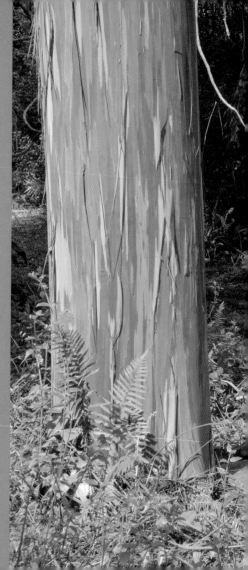

"Patience, strength, beauty. These trees are my teachers – my friends."

- Shavda Young

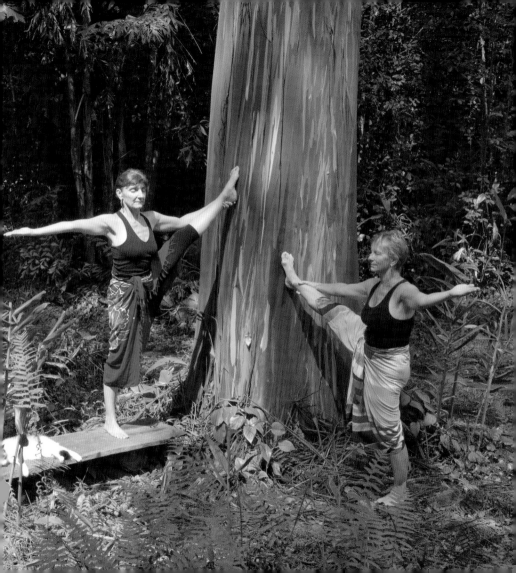

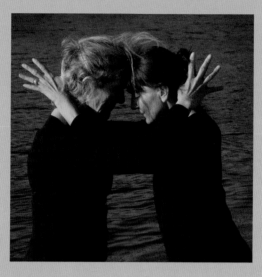

I honor the place in you in which the entire universe dwells. I honor the place in you which is of love, of truth, of light, of peace. When you are in that place in you and I am in that place in me, we are one. Namaste.

- Ancient Salutation

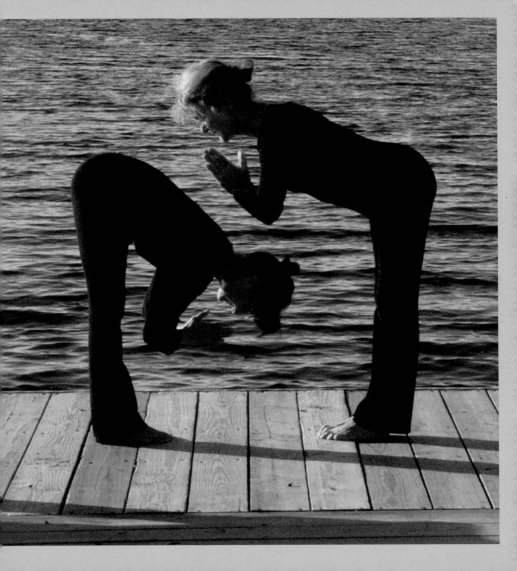

"We stretch. We reach.

We change the world…

together."

~ Sharon Kaufmann

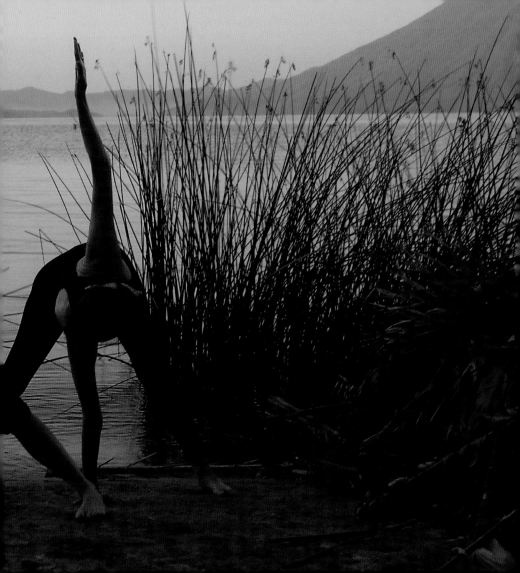

"There are two ways to live your life - one is as though nothing is a miracle, the other is as though everything is a miracle."

- Albert Einstein

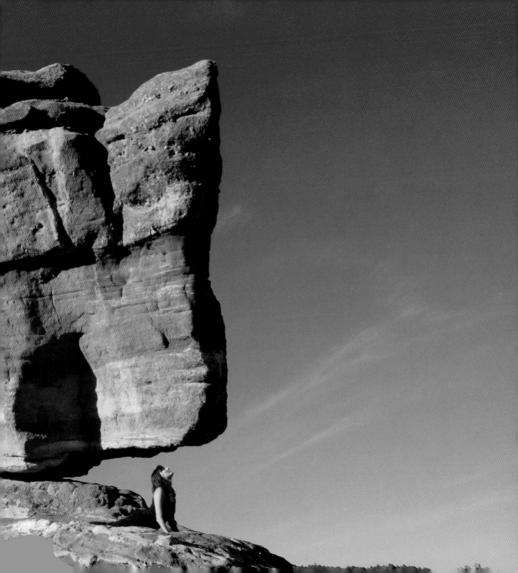

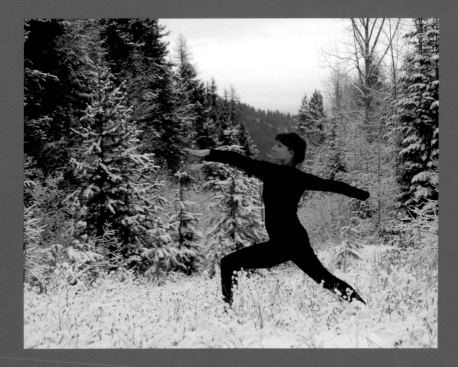

"Friendship with oneself has no season."

- Judith Schwartz

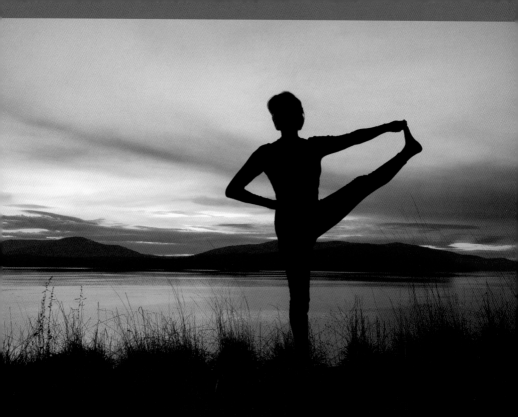

"I want to know if you can be alone with yourself and if you truly like the company you keep in the empty moments."

- Oriah Mountain Dreamer, "The Invitation"

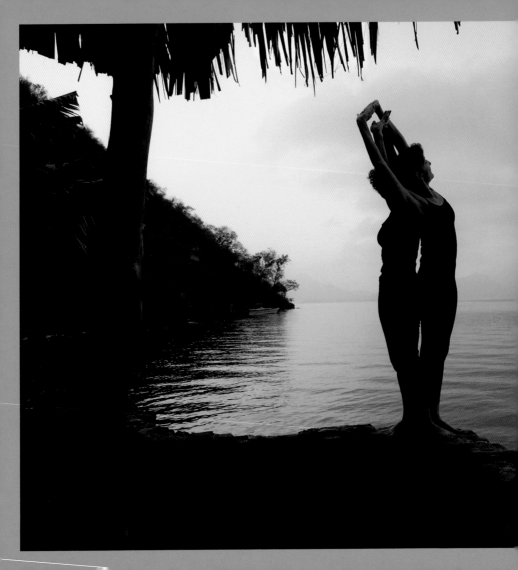

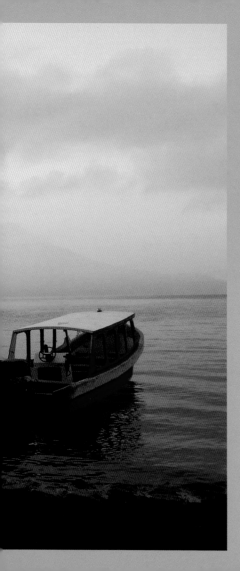

"True friends are created in the heart, not in the world. The world is simply the stage for playing out their love, appreciation and encouragement."

- Kate Gregory

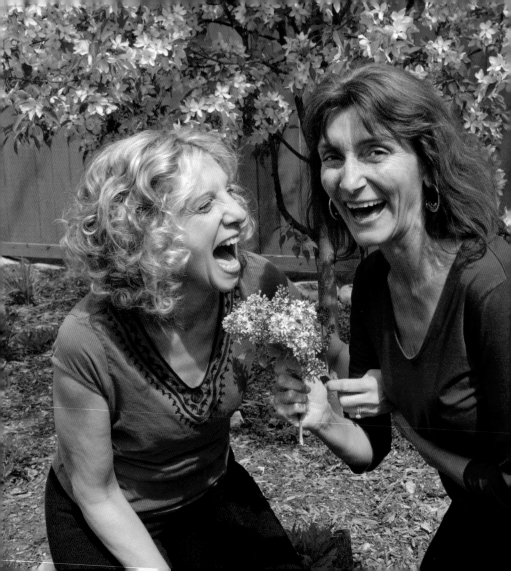

"There is FUN everywhere in life; all you need is to have childlike playfulness at the physical level and playful mental attitude. LAUGHTER YOGA will give you both."

– Dr. Madan Kataria

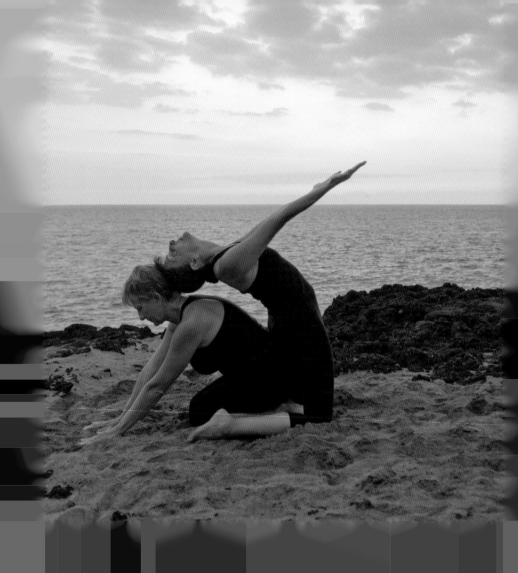

"As you let go of struggle and
relax into the pose, doubts and fears
begin to melt in rivers of acceptance.
The healing flow of love and
compassion is restored."

- Barb Nelson

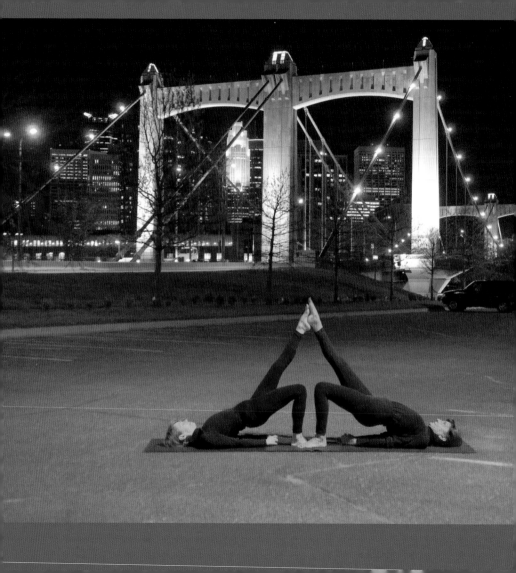

"I cherish the friend that is my bridge to new horizons."

- Lynn Verschoor

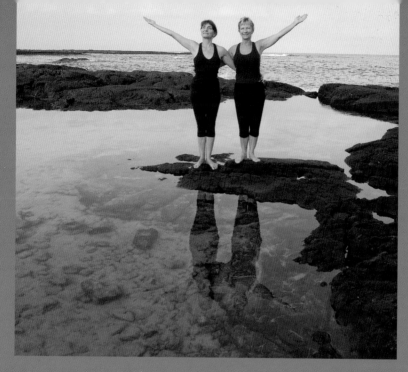

"Everyone and everything that shows up in our life is a reflection of something that is happening inside of us."

— Alan Cohen

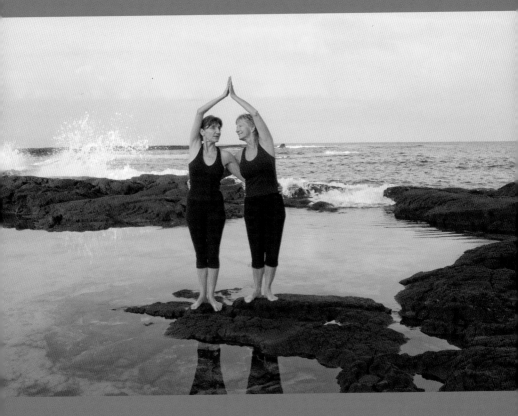

"True friendship is sisterhood of the highest order."

- Lizzie Zielenski

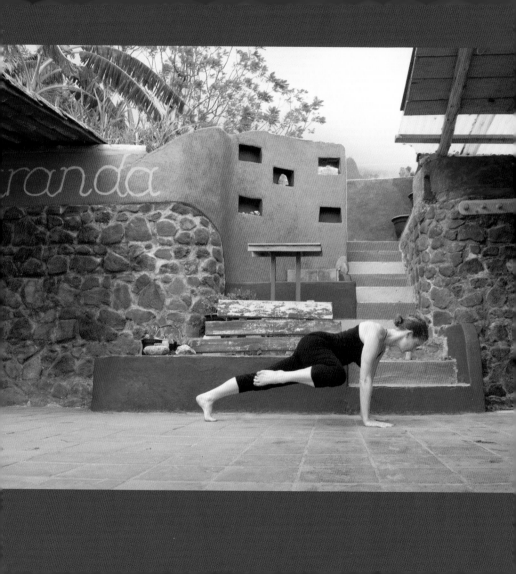

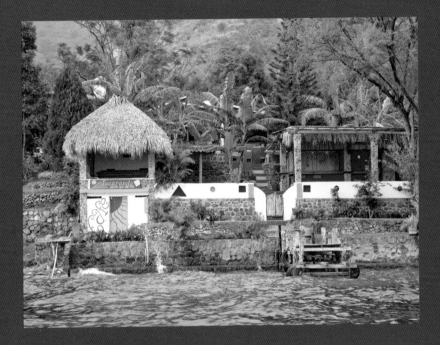

"When life gives you lemons, it's a true friend that will help you to make lemonade."

- Mary Kay McNary

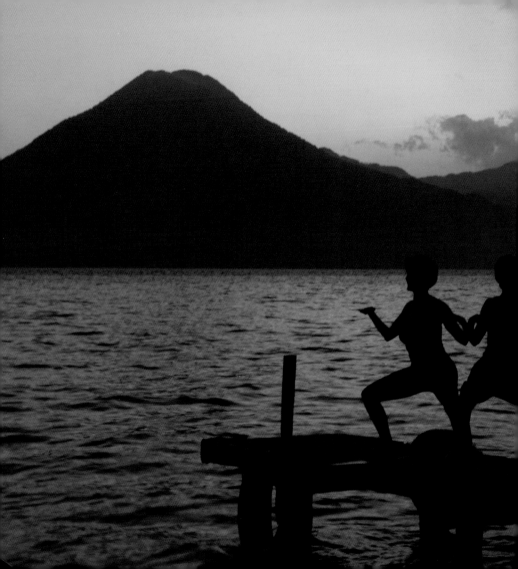

"Each friend represents a world in us, a world possibly not born until they arrive, and it is only in this meeting that a new world is born."

– Anaïs Nin

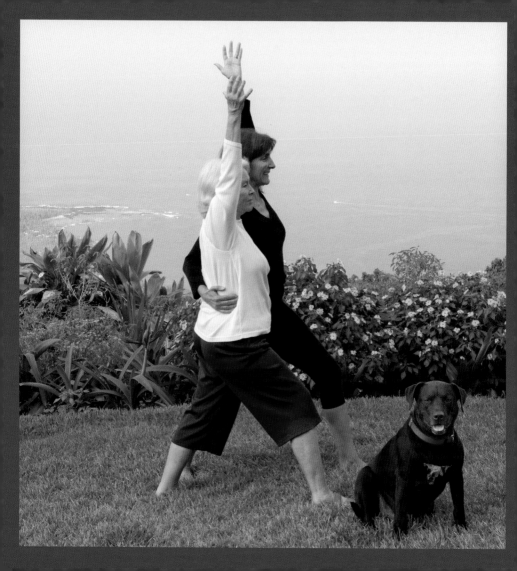

"As we age, friendship is the ability to absorb the meaning of companionship."

– Clara Rischall

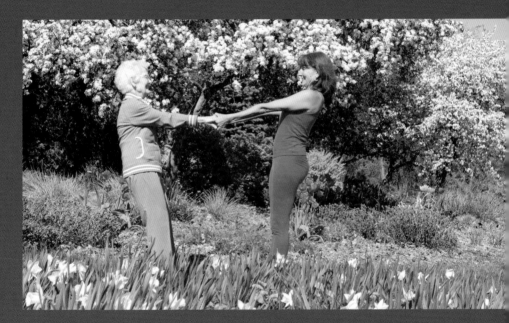

"Friendship and laughter…the fountain of youth."

– Linda Johnson

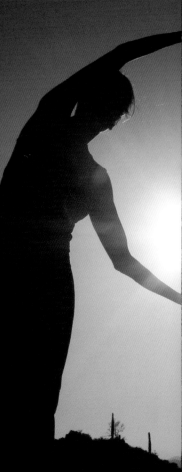

"Friendship is the shadow
of the evening, which
strengthens with
the setting sun of life."

- Jean De La Fontaine

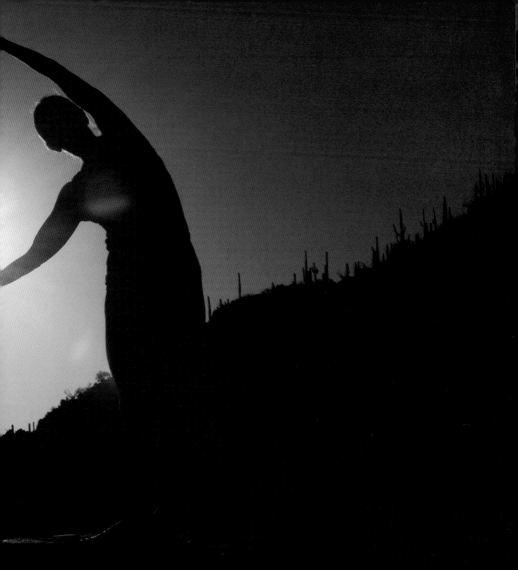

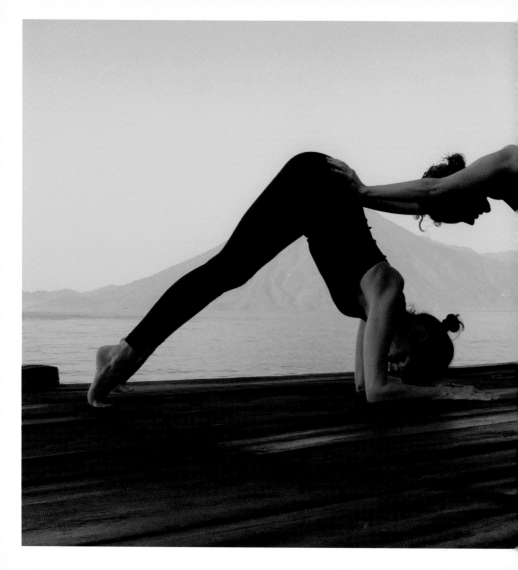

When you are looking for a friend, don't look for perfection, just look for friendship.

- Irish Proverb

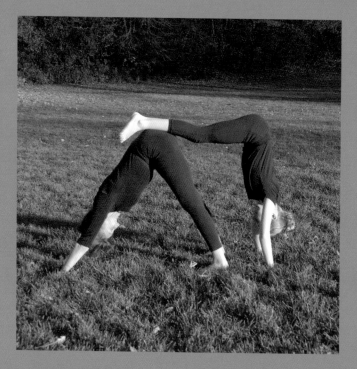

"There is no friendship, no love, like that of the parent and the child."

- Henry Ward Beecher

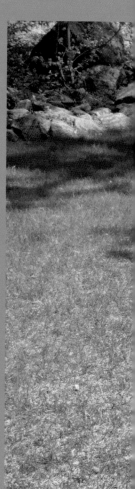

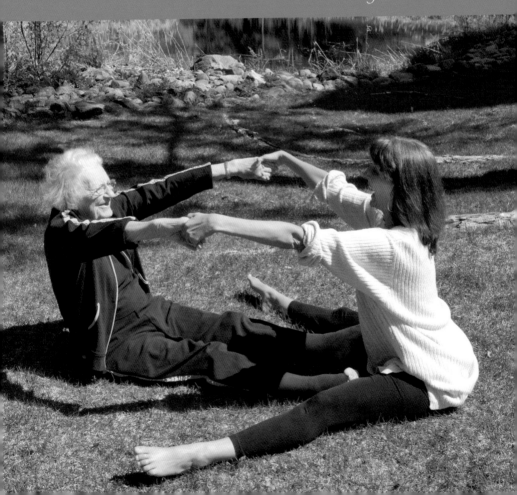

"Age is not important unless you're a cheese."

– Helen Hayes

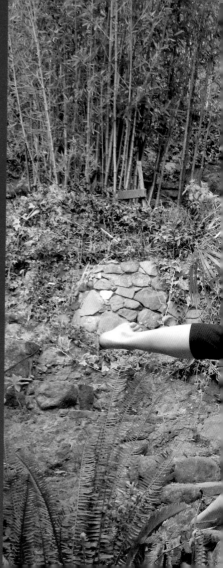

"Some people go to priests; others go to poetry; I to my friends."

~ Virginia Woolf

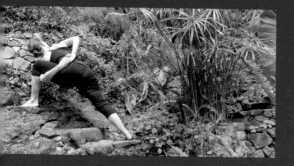

"A true friend will encourage you to grow, and will be there when you falter."

~ Patti Saltzman

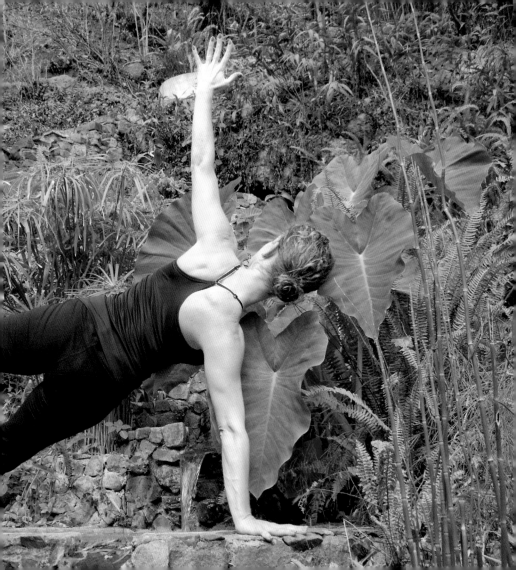

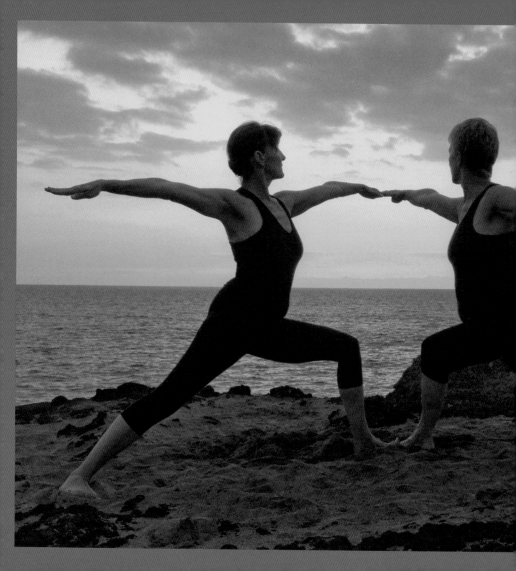

"My dear friend—
she's not so crazy!
Yes, she has her
head in the clouds,
but her feet are
on the ground."

- Valerie Lyon

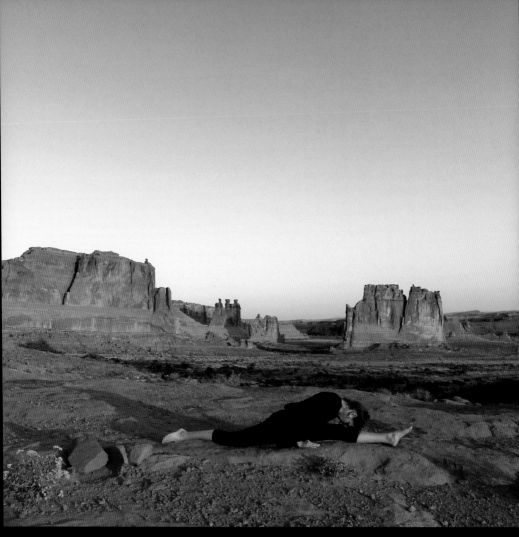

Even the silence holds a sort of prayer.

– Native American Proverb

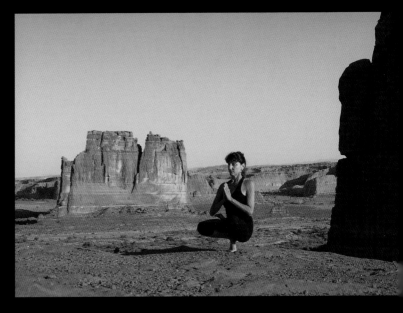

"To dare is to lose one's footing momentarily.

To not dare is to lose one's self."

– Soren Kiekegaard

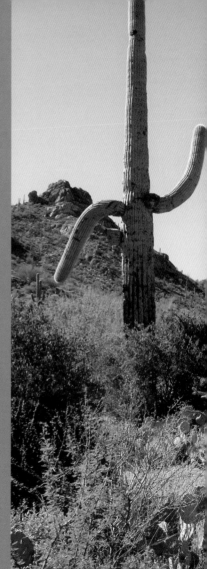

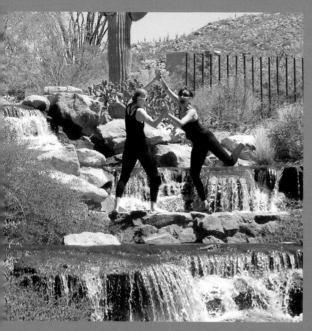

"It is a blessing of
true friends that you
can afford to be
silly with them."

- Ralph Waldo Emerson

"Be careful of the friends you choose
for you will become like them."

- W. Clement Stone

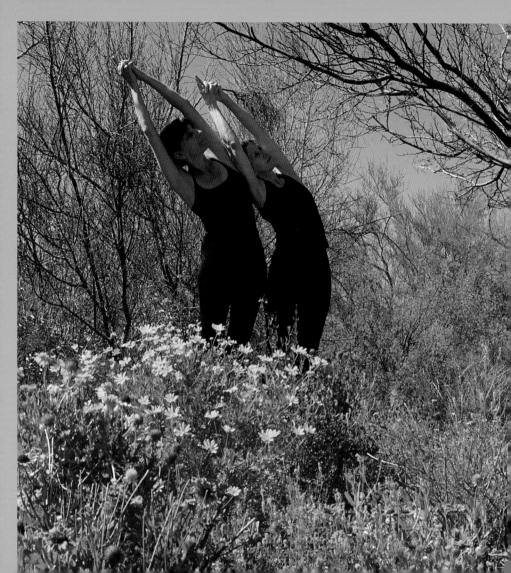

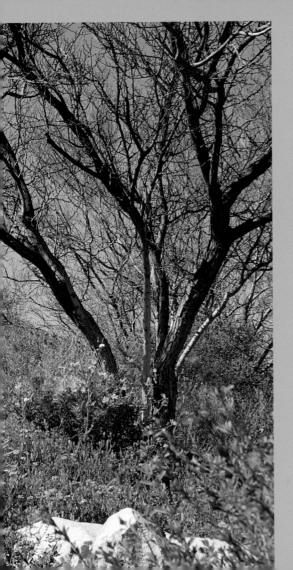

"Be present, my friend.

Listen with an open heart."

- Susan Young

"Friendship is sharing
the view, even when you
see things differently."

- Lynda Austin

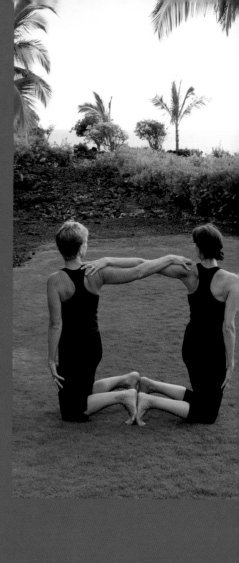

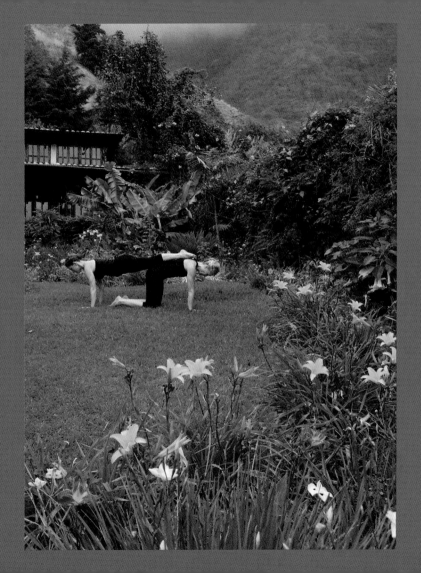

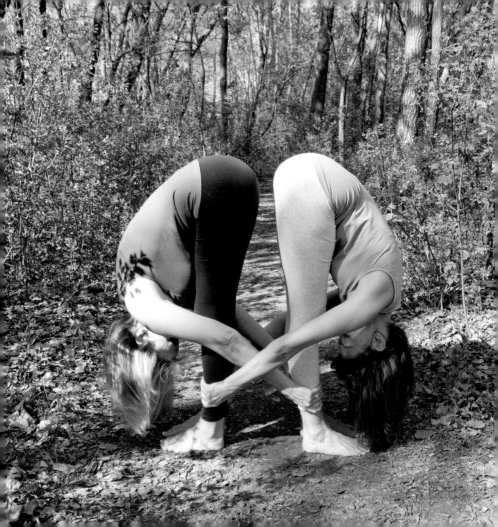

"No ifs, ands or buts…we're on this path together."

– Marlene Johnson

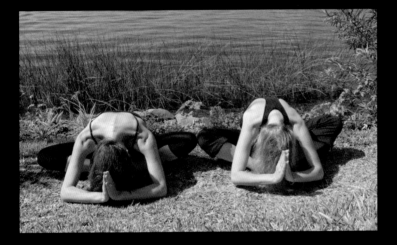

"A good friendship rests solid on any ground."

– Nancy Hammond

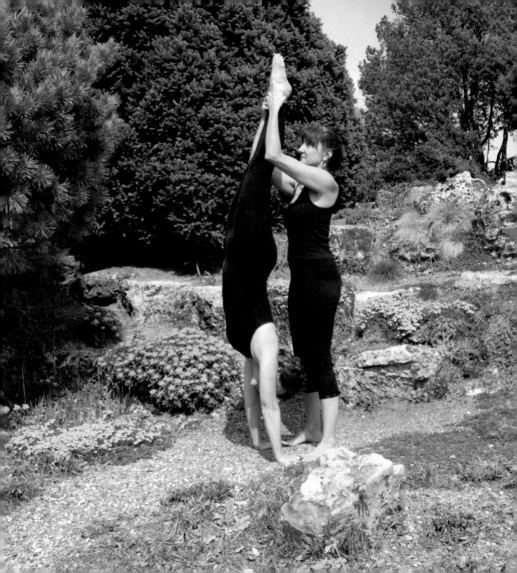

Hold a true friend with both your hands.

- Nigerean Proverb

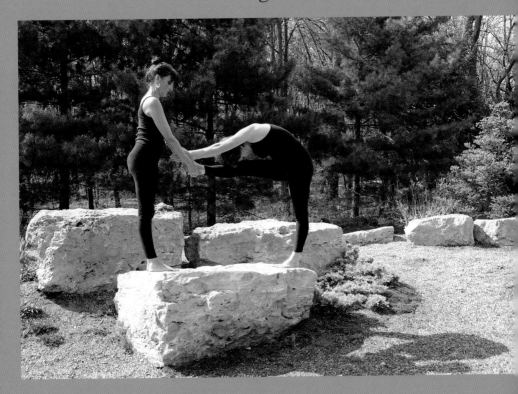

"The best vitamin for making friends, B-1."

- Unknown

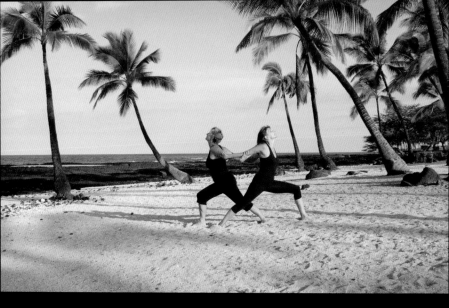

"My courage comes from you my friend."

- Susan Acciani

"I can welcome any challenge with the support of my friend."

- Jill Nicholson

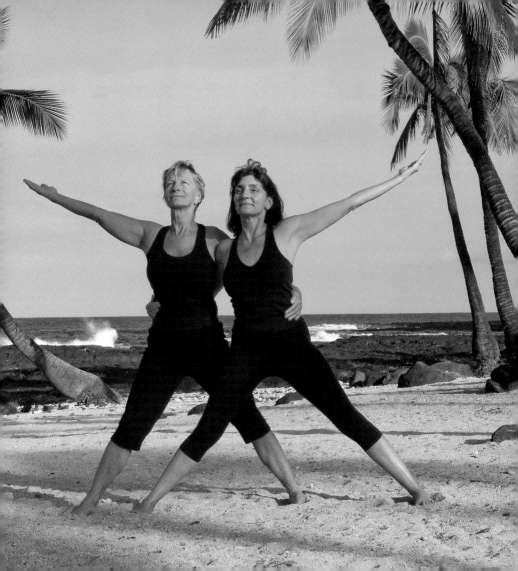

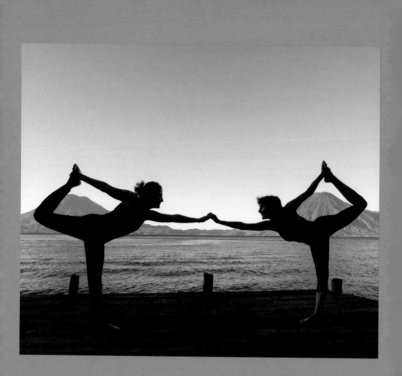

"When you arise in the morning, think of
what a precious privilege it is to be alive
— to breathe, to think, to enjoy, to love."

- Marcus Aurelius

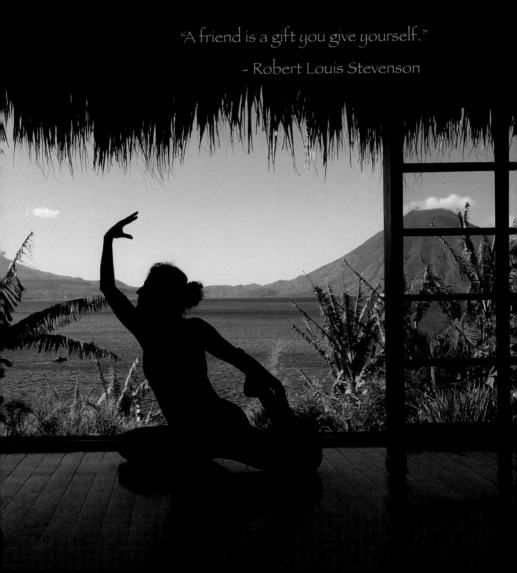

"A friend is a gift you give yourself."

- Robert Louis Stevenson

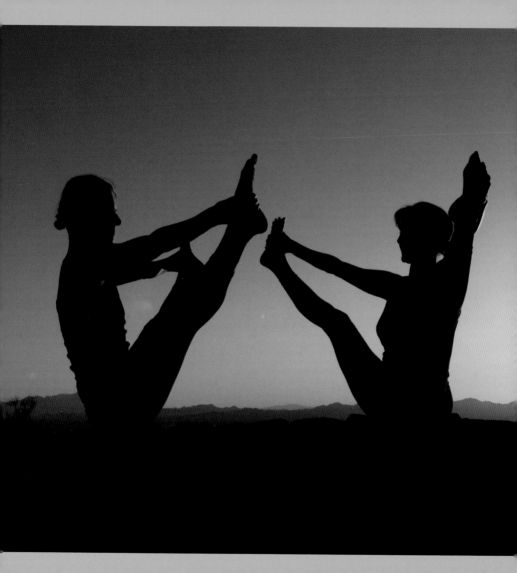

"My core foundation is formed by friends from all walks of life."

- Christine Gresser

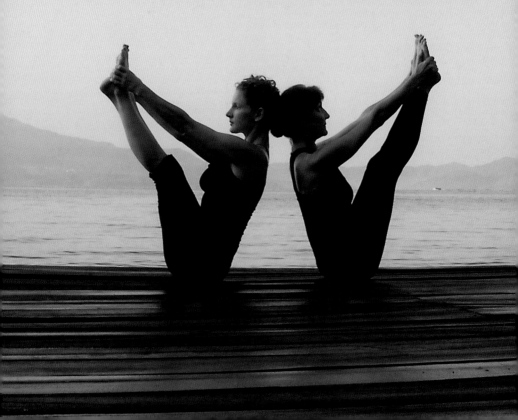

"Never forget the days I spent with you. Continue to be my friend, as you will always find me yours."

– Ludwig Van Beethoven

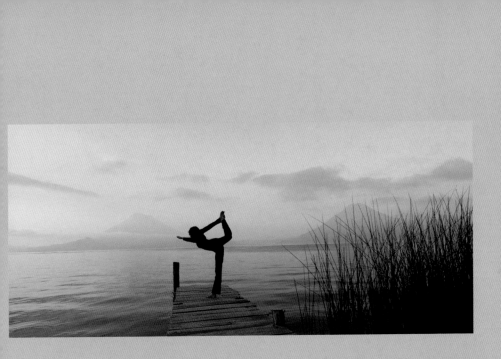

"Friendship with one's self is all important, because without it one cannot be friends with anyone else in the world."

- Eleanor Roosevelt

Acknowledgements

We would like to express our deep appreciation to everyone who offered their camaraderie, laughter and help in creating this book.

A special Thank You to yoginis: Liz Anema, Janet Deming, Anne Fisker, Lucrecia Godoy, Jennifer Gori, Francene Hart, Lyn Kadooka, Diane Kadue, Marcy Lundquist, Claire McNary, Kirsten Mynster, Nēneh Pfeil, Verna Price, Mary Regan, Wendy Stauffer, Evelyn Struthers and J.K. Weber.

Particular appreciation and acknowledgement goes to Russell Kerr for his many talents.

For multiple, supportive ways in bringing this project to fruition we also want to recognize: George Ellis, Richard Britton, Barbara Lee Friedman, James Goodman, Jiten Gori, Diane Kerr, Janet Muehleisen, Jill Nicholson, Jane and Susan Norstrom, Julie Rains, Clara Rischall, Randyl Rupar and Judith Schwartz.

To our amazing, creative publishers: Brett and Sheila Waldman & Bugatti, we offer our utmost respect, heartfelt gratitude and lifetime friendship.

KAHLIL GIBRAN

A Spiritual Treasury

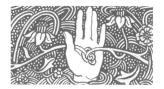

BY KAHLIL GIBRAN

Jesus, the Son of Man

Love Letters

The Prophet

RELATED TITLES PUBLISHED BY ONEWORLD

God's BIG Handbook for the Soul

The Oneworld Book of Prayer

God's BIG Instruction Book

God's BIG Book of Virtues

Words to Comfort, Words to Heal

Rumi: A Spiritual Treasury

KAHLIL GIBRAN

A Spiritual Treasury

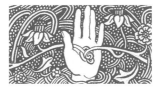

COMPILED BY SUHEIL BUSHRUI

ONEWORLD
OXFORD

KAHLIL GIBRAN: A SPIRITUAL TREASURY

Oneworld Publications
(Sales and Editorial)
185 Banbury Road
Oxford OX2 7AR
England
www.oneworld-publications.com

© Suheil Bushrui 2001
Reprinted 2002

ISBN 1–85168–265–1

Cover and text design by Design Deluxe, Bath
Typeset by Saxon Graphics Ltd, Derby
Printed by Graphicom Srl, Vicenza, Italy

For Jim and Nadia Malarkey
in recognition of their tireless services
to the cause of universal peace.

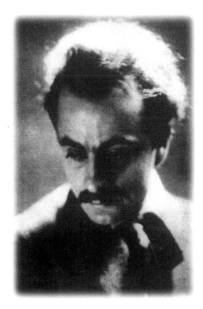

CONTENTS

INTRODUCTION

K AHLIL GIBRAN occupies today a unique position amid the pantheon of the world's great writers and creative geniuses. Long ignored by the literary and artistic establishments of both East and West, who had no convenient niche for a figure such as Gibran who straddled more than one culture, even as his work straddled more than one artistic discipline, his stature and importance have only increased with the passage of time; for although he died in 1931, and his first work was published almost one hundred years ago, his message remains as relevant and urgent today as when it first appeared. With its emphasis on healing and renewal, the universal, the natural, the eternal and the timeless, and its promotion of universal fellowship and the unification of all peoples, his work represents a powerful affirmation of faith in the human spirit.

Inspired by his difficult and, at times, harrowing experiences as an immigrant in an adopted land, he dedicated his life and work to the resolution of cultural and societal conflicts, and in the process developed, as few writers have done before or since, a universal consciousness that transcended the barriers of East and West. In an age that was still rent by internecine strife and world-engulfing conflict, he was a lonely pioneer of conflict resolution, an art which only now is coming into its own.

Gibran's consuming passion, which motivated him in everything he thought and did, was his profound preoccupation with the question of unity, and its achievement in a fragmented world. For Gibran, world unity was not the bland, faceless 'globalization' of the late twentieth century, a melding of diverse cultures into a featureless, indiscriminate blend, but a reconciling and recognition of individual traditions, enabling them to live in harmony together to the mutual benefit of all.

He had an intense foreboding of a world that, in the grip of senseless violence and destruction, was hurtling towards the abyss. Thus it was that, like the hero of his most famous work, he himself assumed almost the role of a prophet, warning mankind of the terrible calamities it would reap from pursuing a path of disunity and anarchy. In his impassioned appeals for unity, his voice rings out as cogently and forcefully at the beginning of the twenty-first century as when he first took up his pen.

In a very real sense, Gibran may be said to embody in himself the successful reconciliation of widely disparate cultures and traditions, languages and literatures. To the casual observer it might appear paradoxical and implausible that a single person should blend within himself influences as diverse as Nietzsche,

Christianity, Islam, the Baha'i faith, the Romantic poets such as Blake and Wordsworth and their contemporaries, and the artistic environments of Paris and New York. Yet he triumphantly achieved this, and in so doing stands as an abiding proof of the viability of such an endeavour, delicate and costly as it was for him, and as it may well be for others; and as a symbol of that unity for which the whole world must now perforce collectively strive – a unity of the very broadest kind, in which the rights of all races, creeds and classes, of women and children, of humankind in general, and indeed of the whole of creation, shall be definitely secured and guaranteed, so that the peoples of the world may be released to lead a new life free from acrimony and conflict.

THIS SPECIAL anthology is in fact a book of spiritual sayings, selected from the writings of Kahlil Gibran. He was a poet of the people writing in 'the book of the people,' expressing in his works the poet's sacred mission of leading us back to the roots of our existence, and renewing in us a sense of the ennobling purpose of our life. Far from erecting a monolithic philosophical system, he expressed his wisdom rather in simple but universal terms that spoke straight to the heart of ordinary people. The unity of purpose informing his artistic vision demanded that his works express a holistic approach to all things, whether relating to the mind, the body or the spirit.

This notwithstanding, it was necessary to devise for this anthology an organizing structure, and for this reason the passages it comprises have been assorted under a selection of titles following for the most part those Gibran himself provided for the sermons of Almustafa in *The Prophet*. Of course, any such principle of arrangement cannot but be inadequate or arbitrary to some degree; but at all events it seemed most appropriate that the anthology should at least reflect the themes of what may justly be accounted his most comprehensive work. To these have been added a few headings reflective of issues that have become pivotal in today's world, such as Human Rights, the Environment, Peace, Religious Harmony, and World Unity.

A S REGARDS the transliteration of Arabic words, I have followed a generally uniform system, except in quoted passages, where the original transliteration has been retained.

American forms of orthography are used only when they occur in quoted passages.

I CAME TO SAY A WORD

MY SPIRIT is to me a companion who comforts me when the days grow heavy upon me; who consoles me when the afflictions of life multiply.

Who is not a companion to his spirit is an enemy to people. And he who seems not in his self a friend dies despairing. For life springs from within a man and comes not from without him.

I came to say a word and I shall utter it. Should death take me ere I give voice, the morrow shall utter it. For the morrow leaves not a secret hidden in the book of the Infinite.

I came to live in the splendour of Love and the light of Beauty.

Behold me then in life; people cannot separate me from my life.

Should they put out my eyes I would listen to the songs of love and the melodies of beauty and gladness. Were they to stop my ears I would find joy in the caress of the breeze compounded of beauty's fragrance and the sweet breaths of lovers.

And if I am denied the air I will live with my spirit; for the spirit is the daughter of love and beauty.

I came to be for all and in all. That which alone I do today shall be proclaimed before the people in days to come.

And what I now say with one tongue, tomorrow will say with many.

A Tear and a Smile

ON GOD

IT IS beautiful to speak of God to man. We cannot fully understand the nature of God because we are not God, but we can make ready our consciousness to understand, and grow through, the visible expressions of God.

Beloved Prophet

WHEN YOU love you should not say, 'God is in my heart,' but rather, 'I am in the heart of God.'

The Prophet

O GREAT intelligent Being! hidden and existing in and for the universe, You can hear me because You are within me and You can see me because You are all-seeing; please drop within my soul a seed of Your wisdom to grow a sapling in Your forest and to give of Your fruit. Amen!

Mirrors of the Soul

T HE SOUL seeks God even as heat seeks height, or water seeks the sea. The power to seek and the desire to seek are the inherent properties of the soul.

And the soul never loses its path, anymore than water runs upward.

All souls will be in God.

Beloved Prophet

THE FIRST thought of God was an angel.
The first word of God was a man.

Sand and Foam

G OD DOES not work evil. He gives us Reason and Learning so that we may ever be on our guard against the pitfalls of Error and Destruction.

The Voice of the Master

O UR GOD in His gracious thirst will drink us all, the dewdrop and the tear.

Sand and Foam

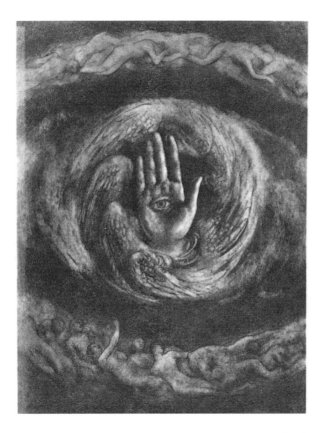

I SEE Him rising like the mist from the seas and the mountains and plains…God is growing through His desire, and man and earth, and all there is upon the earth, rise towards God by the power of desire.

Beloved Prophet

C OMFORT YE, my beloved weak ones, for there is a Great Power behind and beyond this world of Matter, a Power that is all Justice, Mercy, Pity and Love.

The Voice of the Master

N O MAN can reveal to you aught but that which already lies half asleep in the dawning of your knowledge…
And even as each one of you stands alone in God's knowledge, so must each one of you be alone in his knowledge of God and in his understanding of the earth.

The Prophet

I HAVE been here since the beginning, and I shall be until the end of days; for there is no ending to my existence. The human soul is but a part of a burning torch which God separated from Himself at Creation.

The Voice of the Master

T HE IDEA of God is different in every man, and one can never give another his own religion.

Beloved Prophet

Y OU, MAN, would see the world with the eyes of God, and would grasp the secrets of the hereafter by means of human thought. Such is the fruit of ignorance.

The Voice of the Master

A LL SOULS will be in God…
When the soul reaches God it will be conscious that it is in God, and that it is seeking more of itself in being in God, and that God too is growing and seeking and crystallizing.

Beloved Prophet

A ND IF you would know God be not therefore a solver of riddles.

Rather look about you and you shall see Him playing with your children.

And look into space; you shall see Him walking in the cloud, outstretching His arms in the lightning and descending in rain.

You shall see Him smiling in flowers, then rising and waving His hands in trees.

The Prophet

ON RELIGION

I F WE were to do away with the [non-essentials of the] various religions, we would find ourselves united and enjoying one great faith and religion, abounding in brotherhood.

A Treasury

Y OU ARE my brother and I love you.
I love you when you prostrate yourself in your mosque, and kneel in your church, and pray in your synagogue. You and I are sons of one faith – the Spirit. And those that are set up as heads over its many branches are as fingers on the hand of a divinity that points to the Spirit's perfection.

A Tear and a Smile

I S NOT religion all deeds and all reflection,
   And that which is neither deed nor reflection, but a wonder and a surprise ever springing in the soul, even while the hands hew the stone or tend the loom?

Who can separate his faith from his actions, or his belief from his occupations?

Who can spread his hours before him, saying, 'This for God and this for myself; This for my soul, and this other for my body?'

All your hours are wings that beat through space from self to self.

He who wears his morality but as his best garment were better naked.

The wind and the sun will tear no holes in his skin.

And he who defines his conduct by ethics imprisons his songbird in a cage.

The freest song comes not through bars and wires.

And he to whom worshipping is a window, to open but also to shut, has not yet visited the house of his soul whose windows are from dawn to dawn.

The Prophet

Pity the nation that is full of beliefs and empty of religion.

The Garden of the Prophet

Your thought advocates Judaism, Brahmanism, Buddhism, Christianity, and Islam.

In my thoughts there is only one universal religion whose varied paths are but the fingers of the loving hand of the Supreme Being.

Spiritual Sayings

I have hearkened to the teachings of Confucius, and listened to the wisdom of Brahma, and sat beside the Buddha beneath the tree of knowledge.

Behold me now contending with ignorance and unbelieving.

I was upon Sinai when the Lord shewed Himself to Moses. By the Jordan I beheld the Nazarene's miracles. In Medina I heard the words of the Apostle of Arabia.

Behold me now a prisoner of doubt.

A Tear and a Smile

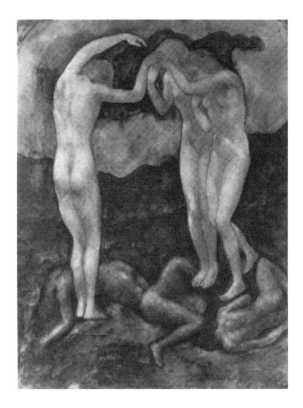

FAITH IS a knowledge within the heart, beyond the reach of proof.

Spiritual Sayings

GOD HAS placed in each soul an apostle to lead us upon the illumined path. Yet many seek life from without, unaware that it is within them.

Spiritual Sayings

RELIGION IS a well-tilled field,
Planted and watered by desire
Of one who longed for Paradise,
Or one who dreaded Hell and Fire.

Aye, were it but for reckoning
At Resurrection, they had not
Worshipped God, nor did repent,
Except to gain a better lot –

As though religion were a phase
Of commerce in their daily trade;
Should they neglect it they would lose –
Or persevering would be paid.

The Procession

GOD MADE Truth with many doors to welcome every believer who knocks on them.

Spiritual Sayings

THERE IS no God but *Allah*...there is nothing but *Allah*. You may speak these words and remain a Christian, for a God Who is good knows of no segregations amongst words or names, and were a God to deny His blessings to those who pursue a different path to eternity, then there is no human who should offer worship.

A Treasury

RELIGION BEGAN when man discerned the sun's compassion on the seeds which he sowed in the earth.

Spiritual Sayings

MANY A doctrine is like a window pane. We see truth through it, but it divides us from truth.

Sand and Foam

SCIENCE AND religion are in full accord, but science and faith are in complete discord.

Spiritual Sayings

MANY TIMES the Christ has come to the world, and He has walked many lands. And always He has been deemed a stranger and a madman.

Jesus, the Son of Man

THE TRULY religious man does not embrace a religion; and he who embraces one has no religion.

Spiritual Sayings

DOUBT IS a pain too lonely to know that faith is his twin brother.

Jesus, the Son of Man

FAITH IS an oasis in the heart which will never be reached by the caravan of thinking.

Sand and Foam

B UT I found it was not a kingdom that Jesus sought, nor was it from the Romans He would have had us free. His kingdom was but the kingdom of the heart.

Jesus, the Son of Man

O NCE EVERY hundred years Jesus of Nazareth meets Jesus of the Christian in a garden among the hills of Lebanon. And they talk long; and each time Jesus of Nazareth goes away saying to Jesus of the Christian, 'My friend, I fear we shall never, never agree.'

Sand and Foam

ON JESUS

HUMANITY LOOKS upon Jesus the Nazarene as a poor-born Who suffered misery and humiliation with all of the weak. And He is pitied, for Humanity believes He was crucified painfully...And all that Humanity offers to Him is crying and wailing and lamentation. For centuries Humanity has been worshipping weakness in the person of the Saviour.

The Nazarene was not weak! He was strong and is strong! But people refuse to heed the true meaning of strength.

The Secrets of the Heart

JESUS WAS not a bird with broken wings; He was a raging tempest who broke all crooked wings. He feared not His persecutors nor His enemies. He suffered not before His killers. Free and brave and daring He was. He defied all despots and oppressors. He saw the contagious pustules and amputated them...He muted Evil and He crushed Falsehood and He choked Treachery.

The Secrets of the Heart

J ESUS NEVER lived a life of fear, nor did He die suffering or complaining ... He lived as a leader; He was crucified as a crusader; He died with a heroism that frightened His killers and tormentors.

The Secrets of the Heart

J ESUS CAME not from the heart of the circle of Light to destroy the homes and build upon their ruins the convents and monasteries. He did not persuade the strong man to become a monk or a priest, but He came to send forth upon this earth a new spirit, with power to crumble the foundation of any monarchy built upon human bones and skulls...He came to demolish the majestic palaces, constructed upon the graves of the weak, and crush the idols, erected upon the bodies of the poor. Jesus was not sent here to teach the people to build magnificent churches and temples amidst the cold wretched huts and dismal hovels...He came to make the human heart a temple, and the soul an altar, and the mind a priest.

These were the missions of Jesus the Nazarene, and these are the teachings for which He was crucified. And if Humanity were wise, she would stand today and sing in strength the song of conquest and the hymn of triumph.

The Secrets of the Heart

'WHO ARE YOU?' I inquired, fearfully, slowly. With a voice that sounded like the roar of the ocean, he thundered, bitterly, 'I am the revolution who builds what the nations destroy…I am the tempest who uproots the plants, grown by the ages…I am the one who came to spread war on earth and not peace, for man is content only in misery!' And, with tears coursing down his cheeks, he stood up high, and a mist of light grew about him, and he stretched forth his arms, and I saw the marks of the nails in the palms of his hands; I prostrated myself before him convulsively and cried out, saying, 'Oh Jesus, the Nazarene!'

The Secrets of the Heart

CHRIST'S DEATH, as well as his life, had a wonderful effect on his followers. The day will come when we shall think but just of the Flame – of the fullness of Life that burned in him…

Christ changed the human mind and for men found a new path.

Beloved Prophet

I N JESUS the elements of our bodies and our dreams came together according to law. All that was timeless before Him became timeful in Him.

They say He gave sight to the blind and walking to the paralyzed, and that He drove devils out of madmen.

Perchance blindness is but a dark thought that can be overcome by a burning thought. Perchance a withered limb is but idleness that can be quickened by energy. And perhaps the devils, these restless elements in our life, are driven out by the angels of peace and serenity.

They say He raised the dead to life. If you can tell me *what is death*, then I will tell you *what is life*.

In a field I have watched an acorn, a thing so still and seemingly useless. And in the spring I have seen that acorn take roots and rise, the beginning of an oak tree, towards the sun.

Surely you would deem this a miracle, yet that miracle is wrought a thousand thousand times in the drowsiness of every autumn and the passion of every spring.

Jesus, the Son of Man

ON LOVE

L OVE IS the only freedom in the world because it so elevates the spirit that the laws of humanity and the phenomena of nature do not alter its course.

The Broken Wings

D RY YOUR tears, my darling, for love that has opened our eyes and made us its servants will grant us the blessing of patience and forbearance. Dry your tears and be consoled, for we have made a covenant with love, and for that love shall we bear the torment of poverty and the bitterness of misfortune and the pain of separation.

A Tear and a Smile

M EN REAP not love save after painful absence and bitter patience and black despair.

A Tear and a Smile

WHEN LOVE beckons to you, follow him,
Though his ways are hard and steep.
And when his wings enfold you yield to him,
Though the sword hidden among his pinions may
    wound you.
And when he speaks to you believe in him,
Though his voice may shatter your dreams as the
    north wind lays waste the garden.
For even as love crowns you so shall he crucify you.
Even as he is for your growth so is he for your pruning.
Even as he ascends to your height and caresses your
    tenderest branches that quiver in the sun,
So shall he descend to your roots and shake them in
    their clinging to the earth.
Like sheaves of corn he gathers you unto himself.
He threshes you to make you naked.
He sifts you to free you from your husks.
He grinds you to whiteness.
He kneads you until you are pliant;
And then he assigns you to his sacred fire, that you may
    become sacred bread for God's sacred feast.

The Prophet

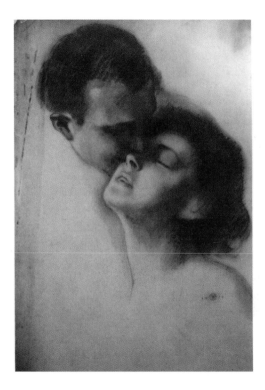

H E PERCEIVED the feathery touch of delicate wings rustling about his flaming heart, and a great love possessing him…A love whose power separates the mind from the world of quantity and measurement…A love that talks when the tongue of Life is muted… A love that stands as a blue beacon to point out the path, guiding with no visible light.

Between Night and Morn

L IFE WITHOUT Love is like a tree without blossom and fruit. And Love without Beauty is like flowers without scent and fruits without seeds…Life, Love, and Beauty are three persons in one, who cannot be separated or changed.

Thoughts and Meditations

IN TRUTH have earthly bodies desires unbeknown
And must they oft-times separate for earthly purpose,
And remain apart for worldly reason.
But all spirits abide in safety in love's hands
Till Death do come and bear them aloft to God.

A Tear and a Smile

TELL ME, for Love's sake, what is that flame which burns in my heart and devours my strength and dissolves my will?

Thoughts and Meditations

IT IS wrong to think that love comes from long companionship and persevering courtship. Love is the offspring of spiritual affinity and unless that affinity is created in a moment, it will not be created in years or even generations.

The Broken Wings

IT IS but the love of a blind man who knows not the beauty of one nor the ugliness of another.

The Forerunner

FOR LOVE when love is homesick exhausts time's measurements and time's soundings.

The Garden of the Prophet

LOVE IS a gracious host to his guests though to the unbidden his house is a mirage and a mockery.

Jesus, the Son of Man

LOVE PASSES by us, robed in meekness; but we flee from her in fear, or hide in the darkness; or else pursue her, to do evil in her name.

The Voice of the Master

LOVE IS a sacred mystery.
To those who love, it remains forever wordless;
But to those who do not love, it may be but a
    heartless jest.

Jesus, the Son of Man

EVEN THE wisest among us bows under the heavy weight of Love; but in truth she is as light as the frolicsome breeze of Lebanon.

The Voice of the Master

LOVE KNOWS not its depth till the hour of separation.

Spiritual Sayings

LOVE IS a word of light, written by a hand of light, upon a page of light.

Sand and Foam

LOVE, LIKE death, changes everything.

Spiritual Sayings

THE FIRST glance from the eyes of the beloved is like the spirit that moved upon the face of the waters, giving birth to heaven and earth, when the Lord spoke and said, 'Let there be.'

The Voice of the Master

WAS THE love of Judas' mother for her son less than the love of Mary for Jesus?

Sand and Foam

WHEN LOVE becomes vast love becomes wordless.

Jesus, the Son of Man

O LOVE, whose lordly hand
Has bridled my desires,
And raised my hunger and my thirst
To dignity and pride,
Let not the strong in me and the constant
Eat the bread or drink the wine
That tempt my weaker self.
Let me rather starve,
And let my heart parch with thirst,
And let me die and perish,
Ere I stretch my hand
To a cup you did not fill,
Or a bowl you did not bless.

The Forerunner

ON MARRIAGE

WILL YOU accept a heart that loves,
But never yields? And burns, but
Never melts? Will you be at ease
With a soul that quivers before the
Tempest, but never surrenders to it?
Will you accept one as a companion
Who makes not slaves, nor will become
One? Will you own me but not possess
Me, by taking my body and not my heart?

The Secrets of the Heart

HER BODY trembled like the trembling of a lily before the breeze of daybreak. The light in her heart overflowed from her eyes, and shyness fought with her tongue for mastery, and she said: 'We are both of us between the hands of a hidden force, a just and merciful force; let it do with us as it will.'

Spirits Rebellious

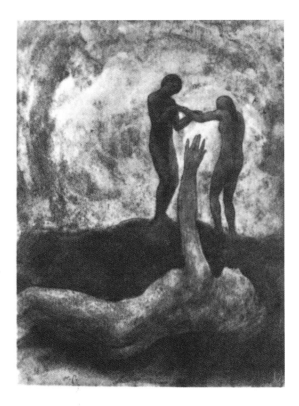

LOVE ONE another, but make not a bond of love:
Let it rather be a moving sea between the shores of
    your souls…
Sing and dance together and be joyous, but let each
    one of you be alone,
Even as the strings of a lute are alone though they
    quiver with the same music.

Give your hearts, but not into each other's keeping.
For only the hand of Life can contain your hearts.
And stand together yet not too near together:
For the pillars of the temple stand apart,
And the oak tree and the cypress grow not in each
    other's shadow.

The Prophet

MARRIAGE IS the union of two divinities that a third might be born on earth. It is the union of two souls in a strong love for the abolishment of separateness. It is the higher unity which fuses the separate unities within the two spirits. It is the golden ring in a chain whose beginning is a glance, and whose ending is Eternity. It is the pure rain that falls from an unblemished sky to fructify and bless the fields of divine Nature.

On Marriage ❧31

As the first glance from the eyes of the beloved is like a seed sown in the human heart, and the first kiss of her lips like a flower upon the branch of the Tree of Life, so the union of two lovers in marriage is like the first fruit of the first flower of that seed.

The Voice of the Master

MARRIAGE IS either death or life; there is no betwixt and between.

Spiritual Sayings

ARE YOU a husband who regards the wrongs he has committed as lawful, but those of his wife as unlawful? If so, you are like those extinct savages who lived in caves and covered their nakedness with hides.

Or are you a faithful companion, whose wife is ever at his side, sharing his every thought, rapture, and victory? If so, you are as one who at dawn walks at the head of a nation toward the high noon of justice, reason and wisdom.

The Voice of the Master

ON WOMEN AND WOMEN'S RIGHTS

FOR OUT of the sensitive heart of a woman comes forth the happiness of mankind, and in the sentiments of her noble spirit are born the sentiments of their spirits.

Spirits Rebellious

MODERN CIVILIZATION has made woman a little wiser, but it has increased her suffering because of man's covetousness. The woman of yesterday was a happy wife, but the woman of today is a miserable mistress.

The Broken Wings

FOR BLIND law and corrupt tradition punish the fallen woman but look tolerantly upon the man.

Spirits Rebellious

MEN WHO do not forgive women their little faults will never enjoy their great virtues.

Sand and Foam

THE MOST beautiful word on the lips of mankind is the word 'Mother', and the most beautiful call is the call of 'My mother'. It is a word full of hope and love, a sweet and kind word coming from the depths of the heart.

The Broken Wings

THEN HE looked at me, and the noontide of His eyes was upon me, and He said: 'You have many lovers, and yet I alone love you. Other men love themselves in your nearness. I love you in your self. Other men see a beauty in you that shall fade away sooner than their own years. But I see in you a beauty that shall not fade away, and in the autumn of your days that beauty shall not be afraid to gaze at itself in the mirror, and it shall not be offended.

'I alone love the unseen in you.'

Jesus, the Son of Man

WOMAN SHALL be forever the womb and the cradle, but never the tomb.

Jesus, the Son of Man

BUT MY dear readers, don't you think that such a woman is like a nation that is oppressed by priests and rulers? Don't you believe that thwarted love which leads a woman to the grave is like the despair which pervades the people of the earth? A woman is to a nation as light is to a lamp. Will not the light be dim if the oil in the lamp is low?

The Broken Wings

IF YOU wish to understand a woman, watch her mouth when she smiles; but to study a man, observe the whiteness of his eyes when he is angry.

Spiritual Sayings

A WOMAN'S heart will not change with time or season; even if it dies eternally, it will never perish.

The Broken Wings

I AM indebted for all that I call 'I' to women, ever since I was an infant. Women opened the windows of my eyes and the doors of my spirit. Had it not been for the woman-mother, the woman-sister, and the woman-friend, I would have been sleeping among those who seek the tranquillity of the world with their snoring.

A Self-Portrait

H E WHO pities woman depreciates her. He who attributes to her the evils of society oppresses her. He who thinks her goodness is of his goodness and her evil of his evil is shameless in his pretensions. But he who accepts her as God made her does her justice.

Spiritual Sayings

T HE POETS and writers are trying to understand the reality of woman, but up to this day they have not understood the hidden secrets of her heart, because they look upon her from behind the sexual veil and see nothing but externals; they look upon her through a magnifying glass of hatefulness and find nothing except weakness and submission.

The Broken Wings

A WOMAN may veil her face with a smile.

Sand and Foam

E VERY MAN loves two women; the one is the creation of his imagination, and the other is not yet born.

Sand and Foam

T HE MAN buys glory and reputation, but the woman pays the price.

The Broken Wings

A Y, MY friend, the spirit descended upon me and blessed me. A great love has made my heart a pure altar. It is woman, my friend – woman that I thought yesterday a toy in the hands of man – who has delivered me from the darkness of hell and opened before me the gates of Paradise where I have entered.

Thoughts and Meditations

MARRIAGE IN these days is a mockery whose management is in the hands of young men and parents. In most countries the young men win while the parents lose. The woman is looked upon as a commodity, purchased and delivered from one house to another. In time her beauty fades and she becomes like an old piece of furniture left in a dark corner.

The Broken Wings

ON CHILDREN

YOUR CHILDREN are not your children.
They are the sons and daughters of Life's longing for
    itself.
They come through you but not from you,
And though they are with you yet they belong not to
    you.

The Prophet

WE OFTEN sing lullabies to our children that we ourselves
may sleep.

Sand and Foam

FOR WOMEN travel not save when led by their
children…Our children do not heed us; like the high tide
of today, they take no counsel with the high tide of
yesterday.

Jesus, the Son of Man

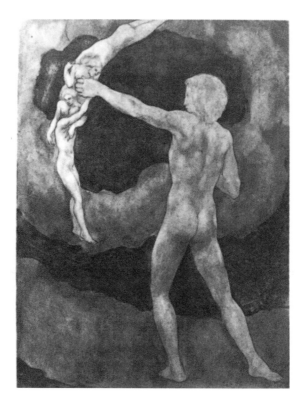

THE SONG that lies silent in the heart of a mother sings upon the lips of her child.

Sand and Foam

THE CALAMITY of the sons lies in the endowments of the parents. And he who does not deny them will remain the slave of Death until he dies.

Spiritual Sayings

SOME OF our children are our justifications and some are but our regrets.

Sand and Foam

THE FOUNDLING is an infant whose mother conceived him between love and faith, and gave birth to him between the fear and frenzy of death. She swaddled him with a living remnant of her heart and placed him at the orphanage gate and departed with her head bent under the heavy burden of her cross. And to complete her tragedy, you and I taunted her: 'What a disgrace, what a disgrace!'

Spiritual Sayings

ON SELF-KNOWLEDGE

AND BETWEEN your knowledge and your understanding there is a secret path which you must needs discover ere you become one with man, and therefore one with yourself.

The Garden of the Prophet

MY SOUL spoke to me and said, 'The lantern which you carry is not yours, and the song that you sing was not composed within your heart, for even if you bear the light, you are not the light, and even if you are a lute fastened with strings, you are not the lute player.'

Thoughts and Meditations

ONLY ONCE have I been made mute. It was when a man asked me, 'Who are you?'

Sand and Foam

THE SOUL is a newly developed element in Nature – and like other elements it has its own inherent properties. Consciousness, desire for more of itself, hunger for that which is beyond itself; these, and others, are the properties of the soul, the highest form of matter.

Beloved Prophet

HOW LONG, my soul, will you continue in lamenting
Whilst yet sensible of my weakness?
Until when will you cry out,
Whilst yet I have naught save the speech of men
To tell therein your dreams?

A Tear and a Smile

YOUR SPIRIT'S life, my brother, is encompassed by loneliness, and were it not for that loneliness and solitude, you would not be *you*, nor would I be *I*. Were it not for this loneliness and solitude, I would come to believe on hearing your voice that it was my voice speaking; or seeing your face, that it was myself looking into a mirror.

The Voice of the Master

OFTENTIMES WE call Life bitter names, but only when we ourselves are bitter and dark. And we deem her empty and unprofitable, but only when the soul goes wandering in desolate places, and the heart is drunken with overmindfulness of self.

The Garden of the Prophet

THE MIND weighs and measures but it is the spirit that reaches the heart of life and embraces the secret; and the seed of the spirit is deathless.

The wind may blow and then cease, and the sea shall swell and then weary, but the heart of life is a sphere quiet and serene, and the star that shines therein is fixed for evermore.

Jesus, the Son of Man

IN THE depths of my spirit is a song no words shall clothe;
A song living in a grain of my heart that will flow not as ink on paper.
It encompasses my feeling with a gossamer cloak,
And will not run as moisture on my tongue.

A Tear and a Smile

THE HUMAN heart cries out for help; the human soul implores us for deliverance; but we do not heed their cries, for we neither hear nor understand. But the man who hears and understands we call mad, and flee from him.

The Voice of the Master

IF THE Milky Way were not within me, how should I have seen it or known it?

Sand and Foam

I DISCOVERED the secret of the sea in meditation upon the dewdrop.

Spiritual Sayings

AND SEEK not the depths of your knowledge with staff or sounding line.
For self is a sea boundless and measureless.

The Prophet

WHO SEES not the kingdom of heaven in this world will not see it in the hereafter.

Spirits Rebellious

On Self-Knowledge 45

I HAVE never agreed with my other self wholly. The truth of the matter seems to lie between us.

Sand and Foam

I F REWARD is the goal of religion, if patriotism serves self-interest, and if education is pursued for advancement, then I would prefer to be a non-believer, a non-patriot, and a humbly ignorant man.

Spiritual Sayings

K NOW YOUR own true worth, and you shall not perish.

The Voice of the Master

T HEY SAY if one understands himself, he understands all people. But I say to you, when one loves people, he learns something about himself.

Spiritual Sayings

Y OU MAY judge others only according to your knowledge of yourself.
Tell me now, who among us is guilty and who is unguilty.

Sand and Foam

MY ENEMY said to me, 'Love your enemy.' And I obeyed him and loved myself.

Spiritual Sayings

A TRAVELLER am I and a navigator, and every day I discover a new region within my soul.

Sand and Foam

EACH DAY look into your conscience and amend your faults; if you fail in this duty you will be untrue to the Knowledge and Reason that are within you.

The Voice of the Master

ON THE DUAL NATURE
OF MAN

ONLY THEN shall you know that the erect and the fallen are but one man standing in twilight between the night of his pygmy-self and the day of his god-self.

The Prophet

IT WAS but yesterday I thought myself a fragment quivering without rhythm in the sphere of life.
   Now I know that I am the sphere, and all life in rhythmic fragments moves within me.

Sand and Foam

THEY SAY to me in their awakening, 'You and the world you live in are but a grain of sand upon the infinite shore of an infinite sea.'
   And in my dream I say to them, 'I am the infinite sea, and all worlds are but grains of sand upon my shore.'

Sand and Foam

TO MEASURE you by your smallest deed is to reckon the
    power of ocean by the frailty of its foam.
To judge you by your failures is to cast blame upon the
    seasons for their inconstancy.

The Prophet

MAN IS two men; one is awake in darkness, the other is asleep in light.

Sand and Foam

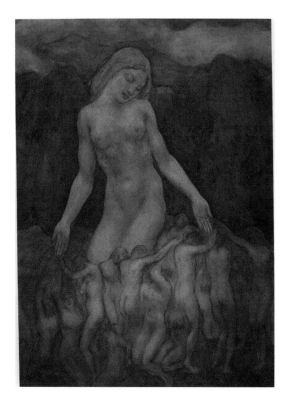

ON IMMORTALITY AND
<u>REINCARNATION</u>

I WAS,
And I am.
So shall I be to the end of Time,
For I am without end.
I have cleft the vast spaces of the Infinite, and taken
    flight in the world of fantasy, and drawn nigh to the
    circle of light on high.
Yet behold me a captive of Matter.

A Tear and a Smile

I AM for ever walking upon these shores,
Betwixt the sand and the foam.
The high tide will erase my footprints,
And the wind will blow away the foam.
But the sea and the shore will remain
For ever.

Sand and Foam

LIKE A pillar of light Man stood amidst the ruins of Babylon, Nineveh, Palmyra and Pompeii, and as he stood he sang the song of Immortality:

Let the Earth take
That which is hers,
For I, Man, have no ending.

The Voice of the Master

ONCE I filled my hand with mist.
Then I opened it, and lo, the mist was a worm.
And I closed and opened my hand again, and behold there was a bird.
And again I closed and opened my hand, and in its hollow stood a man with a sad face, turned upward.
And again I closed my hand, and when I opened it there was naught but mist.
But I heard a song of exceeding sweetness.

Sand and Foam

FORGET NOT that I shall come back to you.
A little while, and my longing shall gather dust and foam for another body.
A little while, a moment of rest upon the wind, and another woman shall bear me.

The Prophet

W E WERE fluttering, wandering, longing creatures a thousand thousand years before the sea and the wind in the forest gave us words.

Sand and Foam

THERE IS not a death in nature,
Nor a grave is set apart;
Should the month of April vanish
'Gifts of joy' do not depart.

Fear of death is a delusion
Harbored in the breast of sages;
He who lives a single Springtime
Is like one who lives for ages.

Give to me the reed and sing thou!
For song is Immortality,
And the plaint of reed remaineth
After the joy and misery.

The Procession

AND HE said to himself:
Shall the day of parting be the day of gathering?
And shall it be said that my eve was in truth my dawn?

The Prophet

H UMANITY IS a river of light running from ex-eternity to
eternity.

Sand and Foam

O MIST, my sister, my sister Mist,
I am one with you now.
No longer am I a self.
The walls have fallen,
And the chains have broken;
I rise to you, a mist,
And together we shall float upon the sea until life's
    second day,
When dawn shall lay you, dewdrops in a garden,
And me a babe upon the breast of a woman.

The Garden of the Prophet

I F IN the twilight of memory we should meet once more, we shall speak again together and you shall sing to me a deeper song.

And if our hands should meet in another dream we shall build another tower in the sky.

The Prophet

I HAVE seen Babylon's strength and Egypt's glory and the greatness of Greece. My eyes cease not upon the smallness and poverty of their works.

I have sat with the witch of Endor and the priests of Assyria and the prophets of Palestine, and I cease not to chant the truth.

I have learned the wisdom that descended on India, and gained mastery over poetry that welled from the Arabian's heart, and hearkened to the music of people from the West.

Yet am I blind and see not; my ears are stopped and I do not hear.

I have borne the harshness of unsatiable conquerors, and felt the oppression of tyrants and the bondage of the powerful.

Yet am I strong to do battle with the days.

All this have I heard and seen, and I am yet a child. In truth shall I hear and see the deeds of youth, and grow old and attain perfection and return to God.

A Tear and a Smile

AND DEATH on earth, to son of earth
Is final, but to him who is
Ethereal, it is but the start
Of triumph certain to be his.

If one embraces dawn in dreams,
He is immortal! Should he sleep
His long night through, he surely fades
Into a sea of slumber deep.

For he who closely hugs the ground
When wide awake will crawl 'til end.
And death, like sea, who braves it light
Will cross it. Weighted will descend.

The Procession

ON LIFE AND DEATH

COME NOW, fair death, for my spirit yearns towards you. Come nigh and loose the fetters of matter, for I am become weary of their dragging. Come then, sweet death, and deliver me from men that reckon me a stranger in their midst because I did speak the tongue of the angels in the language of mankind. Hasten, for men have rejected me and cast me into the corners of forgetfulness because I coveted not wealth as did they, nor profited from him that was weaker than I. Come to me, sweet death, and take me, for those of my kind need me not. Clasp me to your breast, which is full of love; kiss my lips, the lips which tasted not of a mother's kiss, nor touched a sister's cheek, nor felt a sweetheart's mouth. Hasten and embrace me, death, my beloved.

A Tear and a Smile

ONLY LOVE and death change all things.

Sand and Foam

THUS THE nights pass, and we live in unawareness; and the days greet us and embrace us. But we live in constant dread of day and night.

The Voice of the Master

WEAR NOT the black of mourning
But rejoice with me in white raiment.
Speak not in sorrow of my going
But close your eyes and you shall see me among you,
Now and for evermore.
Lay me down upon leafy boughs,
Raise me high upon shoulders,
Then lead me slowly to the wild places.

A Tear and a Smile

WE CLING to the earth, while the gate of the Heart of the Lord stands wide open. We trample upon the bread of Life, while hunger gnaws at our hearts. How good is Life to Man; yet how far removed is Man from Life!

The Voice of the Master

MAYHAP A funeral among men is a wedding feast among the angels.

Sand and Foam

LIFE IS a woman bathing in the tears of her lovers and anointing herself with the blood of her victims.

The Voice of the Master

DRY THEN your tears, my friends,
Raise aloft your heads
As flowers lift up their crowns at dawn's breaking,
And behold Death's bride standing as a pillar of light
Between my bed and the void.
Still your breath awhile and hearken with me
To the fluttering of her wings.

A Tear and a Smile

LIFE IS an enchantress
Who seduces us with her beauty –
But he who knows her wiles
Will flee her enchantments.

The Voice of the Master

I SHALL die now, for my soul has attained its goal. I have finally extended my knowledge to a world beyond the narrow cavern of my birth. This is the design of Life…This is the secret of Existence.

The Secrets of the Heart

THERE, IN the world to come, we shall see and feel all the vibrations of our feelings and the motions of our hearts. We shall understand the meaning of the divinity within us, whom we contemn because we are prompted by Despair.

The Voice of the Master

WE DIE that we may give life unto life even as our fingers spin the thread for the raiment that we shall never wear.

Jesus, the Son of Man

THE REALITY of Life is Life itself, whose beginning is not in the womb, and whose ending is not in the grave. For the years that pass are naught but a moment in eternal life; and the world of matter and all in it is but a dream compared to the awakening which we call the terror of Death.

The Voice of the Master

DEATH IS not nearer to the aged than to the newborn; neither is life.

Sand and Foam

MY SOUL, living is like a courser of the night; the swifter its flight, the nearer the dawn.

The Voice of the Master

ONCE I said to a poet, 'We shall not know your worth until you die.'

And he answered, saying, 'Yes, death is always the revealer. And if indeed you would know my worth, it is that I have more in my heart than upon my tongue, and more in my desire than in my hand.'

Sand and Foam

BECAUSE WE do not understand Life we fear Death, and the fear of Death makes us dread strife and war. Those who *live*, those who know what it is to *be*, those who have knowledge of the Life-in-Death do not preach Peace; *They Preach Life*.

Beloved Prophet

WHEN YOU have solved all the mysteries of life you long for death, for it is but another mystery of life.

Birth and death are the two noblest expressions of bravery.

Sand and Foam

AN OLD man likes to return in memory to the days of his youth like a stranger who longs to go back to his own country. He delights to tell stories of the past like a poet who takes pleasure in reciting his best poem. He lives spiritually in the past because the present passes swiftly, and the future seems to him an approach to the oblivion of the grave.

Broken Wings

YOU WILL be quite friendly with your enemy when you both die.

Sand and Foam

YOUR DAILY life is your temple and your religion. Whenever you enter into it take with you your all.

The Prophet

AFTER SAYING these things he looked about him, and he
   saw the pilot of his ship standing by the helm and
   gazing now at the full sails and now at the distance.
And he said:
Patient, over patient, is the captain of my ship.
The wind blows, and restless are the sails;
Even the rudder begs direction;
Yet quietly my captain awaits my silence.
And these my mariners, who have heard the choir of
   the greater sea, they too have heard me patiently.
Now they shall wait no longer.
I am ready.
The stream has reached the sea, and once more the
   great mother holds her son against her breast.

The Prophet

WHEN LIFE does not find a singer to sing her heart she
produces a philosopher to speak her mind.

Sand and Foam

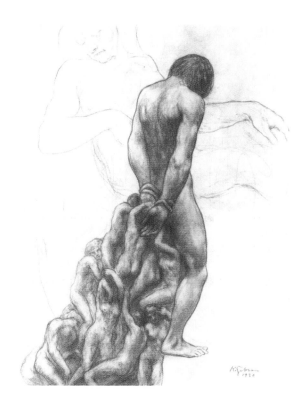

ON HUMAN RIGHTS

Humanity is the spirit of divineness on earth. Divineness walks among the nations speaking of love and pointing to the way of life.

A Tear and a Smile

But I have seen those that covet privilege commend to you the abasement of self the easier to enslave your brothers.

Likewise do they say that the love of existence makes incumbent the robbing of others of their right.

But I say that the protection of another's right is of the noblest and finest of men's acts.

And if my existence be the condition of another's destruction, then, say I, death were sweeter to me.

And if I found no honourable and loving person to kill me, then gladly by my own hand would I bear myself to Eternity before its time.

A Tear and a Smile

THE WISE man is he who loves and reveres God. A man's merit lies in his knowledge and in his deeds, not in his colour, faith, race, or descent. For remember, my friend, the son of a shepherd who possesses knowledge is of greater worth to a nation than the heir to the throne, if he be ignorant. Knowledge is your true patent of nobility, no matter who your father or what your race may be.

The Voice of the Master

I AM KINDLED when I remember the place of my birth, and I lean in longing toward the house wherein I grew; But should a wayfarer seek food and shelter in that house and its inhabitants turn him away, then would my joy be turned to mourning and my longing become a consoling, and I would say:
   'In truth, the house that refuses bread to the needy and a bed to the seeker is most meriting of destruction and ruin.'

A Tear and a Smile

SACRED HUMANITY is the spirit of divinity on earth. That humanity which stands amidst ruins clothing her naked- ness in ragged garments, and shedding abundant tears upon her withered cheeks; calling upon her sons in a voice that fills the air with lament and mourning.

A Tear and a Smile

SPILL MY blood and pierce my body, but you shall not do hurt to my soul neither shall you destroy it. Bind my hands and feet with bonds and cast me into the blackness of a prison cell. Yet you shall not prison my thought, for it is free as the breeze that passes through timeless and boundless space.

A Tear and a Smile

HUMAN SOCIETY has yielded for seventy centuries to corrupted laws until it cannot understand the meaning of the superior and eternal laws.

The Broken Wings

THE SPIRIT deems the power of wisdom and justice above ignorance and tyranny. But it rejects that power which forges out of metal keen-edged swords to spread abroad ignorance and injustice.

A Tear and a Smile

TRUE POWER is a wisdom keeping guard over a just and natural law.

A Tear and a Smile

I YEARN toward my land for its beauty; and I love those that dwell thereon for their weariness.

But did my people take up the sword, saying it was out of love of their land, and fall upon my neighbour's land and plunder its goods and slay its men and render its children orphans and make its women widows, and water its soil with its sons' blood and feed to the prowling beast the flesh of its youth, I would hate my land and its people.

A Tear and a Smile

ON PEACE

L OVE OF self, my brother, creates blind dispute, and disputing begets strife, and strife brings forth authority and power, and these are the cause of struggle and oppression.

A Tear and a Smile

F ROM BEYOND the Future I saw the multitudes prostrate on Nature's breast, turning toward the rising sun, awaiting the morning light – the morning of Truth.

I behold the city razed low, naught remaining of it save its ruins telling of the flight of Darkness before Light…I looked, and beheld not poverty, neither did I see anything above what suffices. Rather did I meet brotherhood and equality.

I saw not any physician, for each morrow is a healer unto itself by the law of knowledge and experience.

Neither did I see a priest, for conscience was become the High Priest.

No lawyer did I behold, for Nature was risen among them as a tribunal recording covenants of amity and fellowship.

A Tear and a Smile

WHAT DESTINY will the giants bring the world at the end of their struggles?

Will the farmer return to his field to sow where Death has planted the bones of the dead?

Will the shepherd pasture his flock on fields mown by the sword?

Will the sheep drink from springs whose waters are stained with blood?

Will the worshipper kneel in a profaned temple at whose altars Satanists have danced?

Will the poet compose his songs under stars veiled in gun smoke?

Will the musician strum his lute in a night whose silence was ravished by terror?

Will the mother at the cradle of her infant, brooding on the perils of tomorrow, be able to sing a lullaby?

Can lovers meet and exchange kisses on battlefields still acrid with bomb fumes?

Will Nisan ever return to earth and dress the earth's wounds with its garment?

Thoughts and Meditations

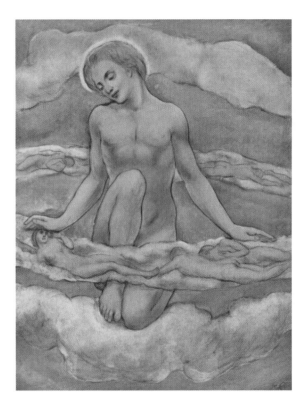

WOULD THAT I could be the peacemaker in your soul, that I might turn the discord and the rivalry of your elements into oneness and melody.

But how shall I, unless you yourselves be also the peacemakers, nay, the lovers of all your elements?

The Prophet

STRIFE IN nature is but disorder longing for order.

Sand and Foam

WHAT IS this duty that separates the lovers, and causes the women to become widows, and the children to become orphans? What is this patriotism which provokes wars and destroys kingdoms through trifles? And what cause can be more than trifling when compared to but one life? What is this duty which invites poor villagers, who are looked upon as nothing by the strong and by the sons of the inherited nobility, to die for the glory of their oppressors? If duty destroys peace among nations, and patriotism disturbs the tranquillity of man's life, then let us say, 'Peace be with duty and patriotism.'

Between Night and Morn

WILL PEACE be on earth while the sons of misery are slaving in the fields to feed the strong and fill the stomachs of the tyrants? Will ever peace come and save them from the clutches of destitution?

What is peace? Is it in the eyes of those infants, nursing upon the dry breasts of their hungry mothers in cold huts? Or is it in the wretched hovels of the hungry who sleep upon hard beds and crave for one bite of the food which the priests and monks feed to their fat pigs?

The Secrets of the Heart

YOU ARE my brother. Why then do you contend with me? Why come you to my land striving to humble me to satisfy them that would seek glory from your words and joy from your labouring?

Why do you forsake your wife and your young to pursue death to a far-off land for the sake of those that lead who would buy honour with your blood and high station with your mother's grief? Is it a noble thing that a man contend in battle with his brother?

Let us raise then an image to Cain and sing the praise of Hanan.

A Tear and a Smile

ON WORLD UNITY AND
THE GLOBAL SOCIETY

I SEE myself a stranger in one land and an alien among one people. Yet all the earth is my homeland and the human family is my tribe. For I have seen that man is weak and divided upon himself. And the earth is narrow and in its folly cuts itself into kingdoms and principalities.

A Tear and a Smile

FOR DEEP in their hearts, though they did not understand it, these nations hungered and thirsted for the supreme teaching that would transcend any to be found on the earth. They yearned for the spirit's freedom that would teach man to rejoice with his neighbour at the light of the sun and the wonder of living. For it is this cherished freedom that brings man close to the Unseen, which he can approach without fear or shame.

The Voice of the Master

EVERY MAN is the descendant of every king and every slave that ever lived.

Sand and Foam

LET US not be particular and sectional. The poet's mind and the scorpion's tail rise in glory from the same earth.

Sand and Foam

YOU ARE my brother and we are the children of one universal holy spirit.

A Tear and a Smile

HE IS of all tribes and yet of none.

Jesus, the Son of Man

IN TRUTH you owe naught to any man. You owe all to all men.

Sand and Foam

AND TAKE with you all men:
For in adoration you cannot fly higher than their hopes
nor humble yourself lower than their despair.

The Prophet

I F YOU would rise but a cubit above race and country and self
you would indeed become godlike.

Sand and Foam

I LOVE MY country with a little of my love for the world, my
homeland;
I love the world with my all, for it is the pastureland of
Man, the spirit of divinity on earth.

A Tear and a Smile

ON ECOLOGY, NATURE
AND THE ENVIRONMENT

NATURE REACHES out to us with welcoming arms, and bids us enjoy her beauty; but we dread her silence and rush into the crowded cities, there to huddle like sheep fleeing from a ferocious wolf.

The Voice of the Master

HOW BEAUTIFUL you are, Earth, and how sublime!
How perfect is your obedience to the light, and how
    noble is your submission to the sun!

How lovely you are, veiled in shadow, and how
    charming your face, masked with obscurity!

How soothing is the song of your dawn, and how harsh
    are the praises of your eventide!
How perfect you are, Earth, and how majestic!

Thoughts and Meditations

TREES ARE poems that the earth writes upon the sky. We fell them down and turn them into paper that we may record our emptiness.

Sand and Foam

AND I heard the brook lamenting like a widow mourning her dead child and I asked, 'Why do you weep, my pure brook?'

And the brook replied, 'Because I am compelled to go to the city where Man contemns me and spurns me for stronger drinks and makes of me a scavenger for his offal, pollutes my purity, and turns my goodness to filth.'

And I heard the birds grieving, and I asked, 'Why do you cry, my beautiful birds?' And one of them flew near, and perched at the tip of a branch and said, 'The sons of Adam will soon come into this field with their deadly weapons and make war upon us as if we were their mortal enemies. We are now taking leave of one another, for we know not which of us will escape the wrath of Man. Death follows us wherever we go.'

Now the sun rose from behind the mountain peaks, and gilded the treetops with coronals. I looked upon this beauty and asked myself, 'Why must Man destroy what Nature has built?'

The Voice of the Master

THOSE OF us who have spent the greater part of our existence in crowded cities know little of the life of the inhabitants of the villages and hamlets tucked away in Lebanon. We are carried along on the current of modern civilization. We have forgotten – or so we tell ourselves – the philosophy of that beautiful and simple life of purity and spiritual cleanliness. If we turned and looked we would see it smiling in the spring; drowsing with the summer sun, harvesting in the autumn, and in the winter at rest; like our mother Nature in all her moods. We are richer in material wealth than those villagers; but their spirit is a nobler spirit than ours. We sow much but reap nothing. But what they sow they also reap. We are the slaves of our appetites; they, the children of their contentment. We drink the cup of life, a liquid clouded with bitterness, despair, fear, weariness. They drink of it clear.

Nymphs of the Valley

AND I knew that the earth is like a beautiful bride who needs no man-made jewels to heighten her loveliness but is content with the green verdure of her fields, and the golden sands of her seashores, and the precious stones on her mountains.

The Voice of the Master

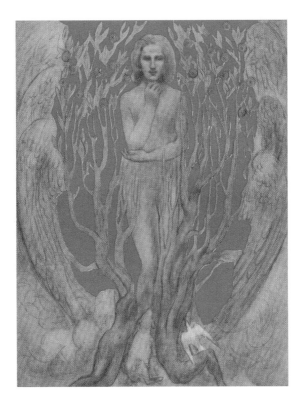

WRATHFULLY AND violently earth comes out of earth; and
    gracefully and majestically earth walks over earth.
Earth from earth, builds palaces and erects towers and
    temples,
And earth weaves on earth, legends, doctrines, and laws.

And earth calls unto earth:
'I am the womb and the sepulchre, and I shall remain a
    womb and a sepulchre until the planets exist no
    more and the sun turns into ashes.'

Thoughts and Meditations

MY GOD-STATE is sustained by the beauty you behold
wheresoever you lift your eyes; a beauty which is
Nature in all her forms. A beauty which is the beginning of the shepherd's happiness as he stands among the hills;
and the villager's in his fields; and the wandering tribes
between mountain and plain. A beauty which is a stepping-
stone for the wise to the throne of living truth.

A Tear and a Smile

THE EARTH breathes, we live; it pauses in breath, we die.

Mirrors of the Soul

EVERY THING in nature bespeaks the mother. The sun is the mother of earth and gives it its nourishment of heat; it never leaves the universe at night until it has put the earth to sleep to the song of the sea and the hymn of birds and brooks. And this earth is the mother of trees and flowers. It produces them, nurses them, and weans them. The trees and flowers become kind mothers of their great fruits and seeds. And the mother, the prototype of all existence, is the eternal spirit, full of beauty and love.

The Broken Wings

WOULD THAT you could live on the fragrance of the earth, and like an air plant be sustained by the light.

But since you must kill to eat, and rob the newly born of its mother's milk to quench your thirst, let it then be an act of worship.

And let your board stand an altar on which the pure and the innocent of forest and plain are sacrificed for that which is purer and still more innocent in man.

The Prophet

SAID A tree to a man, 'My roots are in the deep red earth, and I shall give you of my fruit.'

And the man said to the tree, 'How alike we are. My roots are also deep in the red earth. And the red earth gives you power to bestow upon me of your fruit, and the red earth teaches me to receive from you with thanksgiving.'

The Wanderer

IN MY wanderings I once saw upon an island a man-headed, iron-hoofed monster who ate of the earth and drank of the sea incessantly. And for a long while I watched him. Then I approached him and said, 'Have you never enough; is your hunger never satisfied and your thirst never quenched?'

And he answered saying, 'Yes, I am satisfied, nay, I am weary of eating and drinking; but I am afraid that tomorrow there will be no more earth to eat and no more sea to drink.'

The Forerunner

WHO ARE you, Earth, and what are you?
You are 'I,' Earth…
You are 'I,' Earth.
Had it not been for my being,
You would not have been.

Thoughts and Meditations

On Ecology, Nature and the Environment ⤳ 83

SHALL THERE come a day when man's teacher is nature, and humanity is his book and life his school? Will that day be?

We know not, but we feel the urgency that moves us ever upwards towards a spiritual progress, and that progress is an understanding of the beauty of all creation through the kindness of ourselves and the dissemination of happiness through our love of that beauty.

Nymphs of the Valley

ON THE UNITY OF BEING

M Y SOUL preached to me and showed me that I am neither more than the pygmy, nor less than the giant.

Ere my soul preached to me, I looked upon humanity as two men: one weak, whom I pitied, and the other strong, whom I followed or resisted in defiance.

But now I have learned that I was as both are and made from the same elements. My origin is their origin, my conscience is their conscience, my contention is their contention, and my pilgrimage is their pilgrimage.

If they sin, I am also a sinner. If they do well, I take pride in their well-doing. If they rise, I rise with them. If they stay inert, I share their slothfulness.

Thoughts and Meditations

AND AS a single leaf turns not yellow but with the silent
   knowledge of the whole tree,
So the wrong-doer cannot do wrong without the hidden
   will of you all.

The Prophet

EVERYTHING IN creation exists within you, and everything
in you exists in creation. You are in borderless touch
with the closest things, and, what is more, distance is
not sufficient to separate you from things far away. All things
from the lowest to the loftiest, from the smallest to the greatest,
exist within you as equal things. In one atom are found all the
elements of the earth. One drop of water contains all the
secrets of the oceans. In one motion of the mind are found all
the motions of all the laws of existence.

Spiritual Sayings

FORGIVE ME, my Beloved, for speaking to you in the second
person. For you are my other, beautiful, half, which I
have lacked ever since we emerged from the sacred hand
of God. Forgive me, my Beloved!

The Voice of the Master

WHEN YOU kill a beast say to him in your heart,
'By the same power that slays you, I too am slain; and I
   too shall be consumed.
For the law that delivered you into my hand shall
   deliver me into a mightier hand.
Your blood and my blood is naught but the sap that
   feeds the tree of heaven.'

The Prophet

YOUR MOST radiant garment is of the other person's
   weaving;
Your most savoury meal is that which you eat at the
   other person's table;
Your most comfortable bed is in the other person's
   house.
Now tell me, how can you separate yourself from the
   other person?

Sand and Foam

THE VOICE of life in me cannot reach the ear of life in you;
but let us talk that we may not feel lonely.

Sand and Foam

...AN ATTEMPT to communicate to you that which cannot be communicated to you by anyone other than him who shares in all that is within you. If, therefore, I have fathomed a secret with which you yourself are not unacquainted, then I am one of those to whom Life has granted her gifts and permitted to stand before the White Throne; but if I have fathomed that which is peculiar to me and in myself alone, then let the fire consume this letter.

Love Letters

WE MAY change with the seasons, but the seasons will not change us.

Spiritual Sayings

AND VERILY he will find the roots of the good and the bad, the fruitful and the fruitless, all entwined together in the silent heart of the earth.

The Prophet

FOR IN one soul are contained the hopes and feelings of all Mankind.

The Voice of the Master

I S IT not the hand of God that brought our souls close together before birth and made us prisoners of each other for all the days and nights? Man's life does not commence in the womb and never ends in the grave; and this firmament, full of moonlight and stars, is not deserted by loving souls and intuitive spirits.

The Broken Wings

N OR IS there a single human being with the ability to reshape his dreams, to exchange one image for another, or to transfer his secrets from one place to another. Can what is frail and meagre in us sway the strong and mighty in us? Can the acquired self, earth-bound as it is, induce alteration and transformation in the innate Self, which is of heaven? For that Blue Flame glows immutable, transforms but is not to be transformed, dictates but cannot be dictated to.

Love Letters

AND WHEN you crush an apple with your teeth, say to it in
    your heart,
'Your seeds shall live in my body,
And the buds of your tomorrow shall blossom in my
    heart,
And your fragrance shall be my breath,
And together we shall rejoice through all the seasons.'

The Prophet

THIS EMOTION which we fear and which shakes us when it
passes through our hearts is the law of nature that
guides the moon around the earth and the sun around
God.

The Broken Wings

ON TRUTH

HE WHO listens to truth is not less than he who utters truth.

Sand and Foam

I KNOW faces, because I look through the fabric my own eye weaves, and behold the reality beneath.

The Madman

TRUE LIGHT is that which radiates from within a man. It reveals the secrets of the soul to the soul and lets it rejoice in life, singing in the name of the Spirit. Truth is like the stars, which cannot be seen except beyond the darkness of night. Truth is like all beautiful things in existence: it does not reveal its beauties save to those who have felt the weight of falsehood. Truth is a hidden feeling which teaches us to rejoice in our days and wish to all mankind that rejoicing.

Spirits Rebellious

THE TRUTH that needs proof is only half true.

Spiritual Sayings

IT TAKES two of us to discover truth: one to utter it and one to understand it.

Sand and Foam

I NEVER doubted a truth that needed an explanation unless I found myself having to analyze the explanation.

Spiritual Sayings

A TRUTH is to be known always, to be uttered sometimes.

Sand and Foam

TRUTH IS the will and purpose of God in man.

Spiritual Sayings

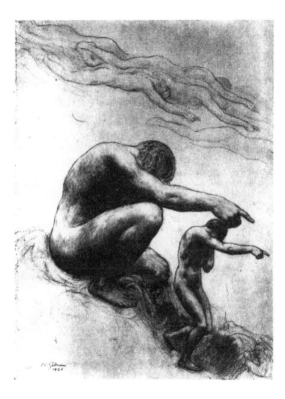

T RUTH CALLS to us, drawn by the innocent laughter of a child, or the kiss of a loved one; but we close the doors of affection in her face and deal with her as with an enemy.

The Voice of the Master

T RUTH IS the daughter of Inspiration; analysis and debate keep the people away from Truth.

Spiritual Sayings

H E WHO would seek Truth and proclaim it to mankind is bound to suffer.

The Voice of the Master

F AITH PERCEIVES Truth sooner than Experience can.

Spiritual Sayings

A N EXAGGERATION is a truth that has lost its temper.

Sand and Foam

I SHALL follow the path to wherever my destiny and my mission for Truth shall take me.

Spiritual Sayings

GREAT TRUTH that transcends Nature does not pass from one being to another by way of human speech. Truth chooses Silence to convey her meaning to loving souls.

The Voice of the Master

I HAVE no enemies, O God, but if I am to have an enemy
Let his strength be equal to mine,
That truth alone may be the victor.

Sand and Foam

SAY NOT, 'I have found the truth,' but rather, 'I have found a truth.'

The Prophet

ON FREEDOM

L IFE WITHOUT Freedom is like a body without a soul, and Freedom without Thought is like a confused spirit... Life, Freedom, and Thought are three-in-one, and are everlasting and never pass away.

Thoughts and Meditations

Y OU ARE free before the sun of the day, and free before the stars of the night;
  And you are free when there is no sun and no moon and no star.
  You are even free when you close your eyes upon all there is.
  But you are a slave to him whom you love because you love him.
  And a slave to him who loves you because he loves you.

Sand and Foam

WE SIT on a high rock and gaze at the distant horizon. She points to the golden cloud; and makes me aware of the song the birds sing before they retire for the night, thanking the Lord for the gift of freedom and peace.

The Voice of the Master

BEYOND THIS burdened self lives my freer self; and to him my dreams are a battle fought in twilight and my desires the rattling of bones.

Too young am I and too outraged to be my freer self.

And how shall I become my freer self unless I slay my burdened selves, or unless all men become free?

How shall my leaves fly singing upon the wind unless my roots shall wither in the dark?

How shall the eagle in me soar against the sun until my fledglings leave the nest which I with my own beak have built for them?

The Forerunner

AND I have found both freedom and safety in my madness; the freedom of loneliness and the safety from being understood, for those who understand us enslave something in us.

The Madman

FREEDOM BIDS us to her table where we may partake of her savoury food and rich wine; but when we sit down at her board, we eat ravenously and glut ourselves.

The Voice of the Master

THEY TELL me: If you see a slave sleeping, do not wake him lest he be dreaming of freedom.

I tell them: If you see a slave sleeping, wake him and explain to him freedom.

Mirrors of the Soul

THE FREEDOM of the one who boasts of it is a slavery.

Spiritual Sayings

WE ARE all prisoners, but some of us are in cells with windows and some without.

Sand and Foam

WE DEMAND freedom of speech and freedom of the press, although we have nothing to say and nothing worth printing.

Spiritual Sayings

GOD HAS given you a spirit with wings on which to soar into the spacious firmament of Love and Freedom. Is it not pitiful then that you cut your wings with your own hands and suffer your soul to crawl like an insect upon the earth?

The Voice of the Master

AND THUS your freedom when it loses its fetters becomes itself the fetter of a greater freedom.

The Prophet

FOR YOU can only be free when even the desire of seeking freedom becomes a harness to you, and when you cease to speak of freedom as a goal and a fulfilment.
You shall be free indeed when your days are not without a care nor your nights without a want and a grief,
But rather when these things girdle your life and yet you rise above them naked and unbound.

The Prophet

THE TRULY free man is he who bears the load of the bond slave patiently.

Sand and Foam

FORGETFULNESS IS a form of freedom.

Sand and Foam

ON GOOD AND EVIL

H E WHO can put his finger upon that which divides good from evil is he who can touch the very hem of the garment of God.

Sand and Foam

T HE GOOD God and the Evil God met on the mountain top.

The Good God said, 'Good day to you, brother.'

The Evil God made no answer.

And the Good God said, 'You are in a bad humour today.'

'Yes,' said the Evil God, 'for of late I have been often mistaken for you, called by your name, and treated as if I were you, and it ill-pleases me.'

And the Good God said, 'But I too have been mistaken for you and called by your name.'

The Evil God walked away cursing the stupidity of man.

The Madman

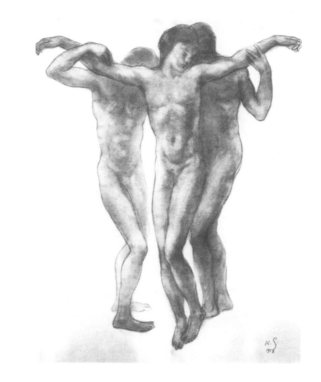

BEHOLD THE sun rising from out of darkness.

A Tear and a Smile

EVIL IS an unfit creature, laggard in obeying the law of the continuity of fitness.

Spiritual Sayings

IF ALL they say of good and evil were true, then my life is but one long crime.

Sand and Foam

WICKEDNESS IS indeed a force to rival goodness in its power and influence.

Love Letters

IF YOU choose between two evils, let your choice fall on the obvious rather than the hidden, even though the first appears greater than the second.

Spiritual Sayings

THE GOOD in man should freely flow,
As evil lives beyond the grave;
While Time with fingers moves the pawns
Awhile, then breaks the knight and knave.

The Procession

EVERY DRAGON gives birth to a St George who slays it.

Sand and Foam

HE WHO does not see the angels and devils in the beauty
and malice of life will be far removed from knowledge,
and his spirit will be empty of affection.

The Broken Wings

ON REASON AND PASSION

WHEN REASON speaks to you, hearken to what she says, and you shall be saved. Make good use of her utterances, and you shall be as one armed. For the Lord has given you no better guide than Reason, no stronger arm than Reason. When Reason speaks to your inmost self, you are proof against Desire. For Reason is a prudent minister, a loyal guide, and a wise counsellor. Reason is light in darkness, as anger is darkness amidst light. Be wise – let Reason, not Impulse, be your guide.

The Voice of the Master

LIFE IS that which we see and experience through the spirit; but the world around us we come to know through our understanding and reason. And such knowledge brings us great joy or sorrow.

The Voice of the Master

YOUR REASON and your passion are the rudder and the sails of your seafaring soul.

If either your sails or your rudder be broken, you can but toss and drift, or else be held at a standstill in mid-seas.

For reason, ruling alone, is a force confining; and passion, unattended, is a flame that burns to its own destruction.

Therefore let your soul exalt your reason to the height of passion, that it may sing;

And let it direct your passion with reason, that your passion may live through its own daily resurrection, and like the phoenix rise above its own ashes.

The Prophet

KEEP A watchful eye over yourself as if you were your own enemy; for you cannot learn to govern yourself, unless you first learn to govern your own passions and obey the dictates of your conscience.

The Voice of the Master

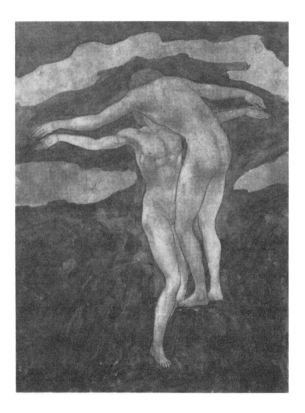

WHERE CAN I find a man governed by reason instead of habits and urges?

Spiritual Sayings

MAKE HASTE slowly, and do not be slothful when opportunity beckons. Thus you will avoid grave errors.

The Voice of the Master

REASON IS not like the goods sold in the market places – the more plentiful they are, the less they are worth. Reason's worth waxes with her abundance. But were she sold in the market, it is only the wise man who would understand her true value.

The Voice of the Master

ON PAIN AND PLEASURE

H OW SHALL **my heart be unsealed unless it be broken?**

Sand and Foam

PLEASURE IS **a freedom-song,**
But it is not freedom.
It is the blossoming of your desires,
But it is not their fruit.
It is a depth calling unto a height,
But it is not the deep nor the high.
It is the caged taking wing,
But it is not space encompassed.
Ay, in very truth, pleasure is a freedom-song.
And I fain would have you sing it with fullness of heart;
   yet I would not have you lose your hearts in the
   singing.

The Prophet

THE PAIN that accompanies love, invention, and responsibility also gives delight.

Spiritual Sayings

THEY SAY the nightingale pierces his bosom with a thorn when he sings a love song.
  So do we all. How else should we sing?

Sand and Foam

LAST NIGHT I invented a new pleasure, and as I was giving it the first trial an angel and a devil came rushing toward my house. They met at my door and fought with each other over my newly created pleasure; the one crying, 'It is a sin!' – the other, 'It is a virtue!'

The Madman

STRANGE, THE desire for certain pleasures is a part of my pain.

Sand and Foam

SAID ONE oyster to a neighbouring oyster, 'I have a very great pain within me. It is heavy and round and I am in distress.'

And the other oyster replied with haughty complacence, 'Praise be to the heavens and to the sea, I have no pain within me. I am well and whole both within and without.'

At that moment a crab was passing by and heard the two oysters, and he said to the one who was well and whole both within and without, 'Yes, you are well and whole; but the pain that your neighbour bears is a pearl of exceeding beauty.'

The Wanderer

A THOUSAND years ago my neighbour said to me, 'I hate life, for it is naught but a thing of pain.'

And yesterday I passed by a cemetery and saw life dancing upon his grave.

Sand and Foam

HAD IT not been for the presence of calamities, work and struggle would not have existed, and life would have been cold, barren and boresome.

A Self-Portrait

THE CRUEL tasks for which we received no reward will live with us, and show forth in splendour, and declare our glory; and the hardships we have sustained shall be as a wreath of laurel on our honoured heads.

The Voice of the Master

A PEARL is a temple built by pain around a grain of sand. What longing built our bodies and around what grains?

Sand and Foam

MUCH OF your pain is self-chosen.
It is the bitter potion by which the physician within you heals your sick self.
Therefore trust the physician, and drink his remedy in silence and tranquillity:
For his hand, though heavy and hard, is guided by the tender hand of the Unseen,
And the cup he brings, though it burn your lips, has been fashioned of the clay which the Potter has moistened with His own sacred tears.

The Prophet

ON CRIME AND PUNISHMENT

VERILY NO crime is committed by one man or one woman.
All crimes are committed by all.

Jesus, the Son of Man

CEASE THIS recital of things forbidden,
For my conscience is a tribunal
That will judge me with justice.
It will guard me from punishment if I am innocent
And withhold from me favour when I am guilty.

A Tear and a Smile

IF THERE is such a thing as sin, some of us commit it
backward following our forefathers' footsteps;
And some of us commit it forward by overruling our
children.

Sand and Foam

I T IS when your spirit goes wandering upon the wind, That you, alone and unguarded, commit a wrong unto others and therefore unto yourself.

And for that wrong committed must you knock and wait a while unheeded at the gate of the blessed...

Oftentimes have I heard you speak of one who commits a wrong as though he were not one of you, but a stranger unto you and an intruder upon your world.

But I say that even as the holy and the righteous cannot rise beyond the highest which is in each one of you,

So the wicked and the weak cannot fall lower than the lowest which is in you also...

Like a procession you walk together towards your god-self.

You are the way and the wayfarers.

And when one of you falls down he falls for those behind him, a caution against the stumbling stone.

Ay, and he falls for those ahead of him, who though faster and surer of foot, yet removed not the stumbling stone.

The Prophet

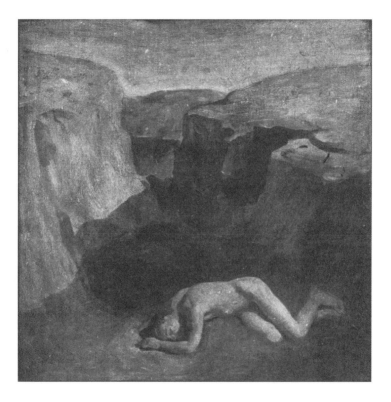

H E WHO forgives you for a sin you have not committed forgives himself for his own crime.

Spiritual Sayings

C RIME IS either another name of need or an aspect of a disease.

Sand and Foam

ON LAWS

ALL THAT is on earth lives by the law of its nature, and by the nature of its law are spread the glories and joys of liberty. But man alone is forbidden this bliss, for he makes earthly laws binding to his mortal spirit, and on his body and soul passes harsh judgement, and raises up about his love and yearning dark prison walls, and for his heart and mind digs a deep grave.

Spirits Rebellious

ONLY AN idiot and a genius break man-made laws; and they are the nearest to the heart of God.

Sand and Foam

EVEN THE laws of Life obey Life's laws.

Spiritual Sayings

JUSTICE ON earth would cause the Jinn
To cry at misuse of the word,
And were the dead to witness it,
They'd mock at fairness in this world.

Yea, death and prison we mete out
To small offenders of the laws,
While honour, wealth, and full respect
On greater pirates we bestow.

To steal a flower we call mean,
To rob a field is chivalry;
Who kills the body he must die,
Who kills the spirit he goes free.

The Procession

I DO not love man-made laws and I abhor the traditions that
our ancestors left us. This hatred is the fruit of my love for
the sacred and spiritual kindness which should be the
source of every law upon the earth, for kindness is the shadow
of God in man.

A Self-Portrait

YOU DELIGHT in laying down laws,
Yet you delight more in breaking them.
Like children playing by the ocean who build sand-
    towers with constancy and then destroy them with
    laughter.
But while you build your sand-towers the ocean brings
    more sand to the shore,
And when you destroy them the ocean laughs with you.
Verily the ocean laughs always with the innocent.

The Prophet

THERE ARE four things a ruler should banish from his
realm: Wrath, Avarice, Falsehood, and Violence.

The Voice of the Master

IT IS the mind in us that yields to the laws made by us, but
never the spirit in us.

Sand and Foam

ON WORK

A ND WHEN you work with love you bind yourself to yourself, and to one another, and to God.

The Prophet

YOU WORK that you may keep pace with the earth and the soul of the earth.

For to be idle is to become a stranger unto the seasons, and to step out of life's procession, that marches in majesty and proud submission towards the infinite.

The Prophet

A LITTLE knowledge that *acts* is worth infinitely more than much knowledge that is idle.

The Voice of the Master

WORK IS love made visible.

The Prophet

THE MASTER knew no rest except in work. He loved work, which he defined as *Visible Love*.

The Voice of the Master

AMBITION IS a sort of work.

Spiritual Sayings

ON GIVING

GENEROSITY IS not in giving me that which I need more than you do, but it is in giving me that which you need more than I do.

Sand and Foam

STRENGTH SOWS within the depths of my heart and I harvest and gather ears of corn and give it in sheaves to the hungry.

The spirit revives this small vine and I press its grapes and give the thirsty to drink.

Heaven fills this lamp with oil and I kindle it and place it by the window of my house for those that pass by night.

I do these things because I live by them, and were the days to forbid me and the nights stay my hand, I would seek death; for death is more meet to a prophet cast out by his nation and a poet who is an exile in his own land.

A Tear and a Smile

THE ONE who receives is not mindful, but the one who gives bears the burden of cautioning himself that it is with a view to brotherly love, and toward friendly aid, and not to self-esteem.

The Secrets of the Heart

THOSE WHO give you a serpent when you ask for a fish may have nothing but serpents to give. It is then generosity on their part.

Sand and Foam

ONCE THERE lived a man who had a valleyful of needles. And one day the mother of Jesus came to him and said: 'Friend, my son's garment is torn and I must needs mend it before he goeth to the temple. Wouldst thou not give me a needle?'

And he gave her not a needle, but he gave her a learned discourse on Giving and Taking to carry to her son before he should go to the temple.

The Madman

HOW MEAN am I when life gives me gold and I give you silver, and yet I deem myself generous.

Sand and Foam

AND NOW let me speak of other things. On a day when He and I were alone walking in a field, we were both hungry, and we came to a wild apple tree.

There were only two apples hanging on the bough.

And He held the trunk of the tree with His arm and shook it, and the two apples fell down.

He picked them both up and gave one to me. The other He held in His hand.

In my hunger I ate the apple, and I ate it fast.

Then I looked at Him and I saw that He still held the other apple in His hand.

And He gave it to me saying: 'Eat this also.'

And I took the apple, and in my shameless hunger I ate it.

And as we walked on I looked upon His face…

He had given me the two apples. And I knew He was hungry even as I was hungry.

But I now know that in giving them to me He had been satisfied.

Jesus, the Son of Man

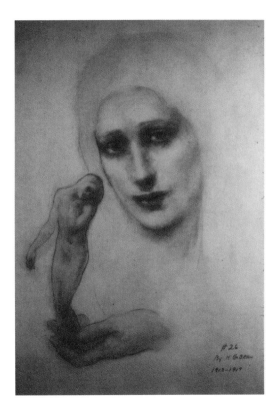

#26
By K GIBRAN
1913-1917

YOU ARE indeed charitable when you give, and while giving turn your face away so that you may not see the shyness of the receiver.

Sand and Foam

YOU ARE good when you strive to give of yourself.

The Prophet

YOU CANNOT consume beyond your appetite. The other half of the loaf belongs to the other person, and there should remain a little bread for the chance guest.

Sand and Foam

THEY GIVE that they may live, for to withhold is to perish.

The Prophet

GENEROSITY IS giving more than you can, and pride is taking less than you need.

Sand and Foam

ON TEACHING AND EDUCATION

I HAVE learned silence from the talkative, toleration from the intolerant, and kindness from the unkind; yet, strange, I am ungrateful to these teachers.

Sand and Foam

LEARNING NOURISHES the seed but it gives you no seed of its own.

Mirrors of the Soul

EDUCATION SOWS not seeds in you, but makes your seeds grow.

Spiritual Sayings

THE TEACHER who walks in the shadow of the temple, among his followers, gives not of his wisdom but rather of his faith and his lovingness.

The Prophet

ARE YOU a teacher standing upon the raised stage of history, who, inspired by the glories of the past, preaches to mankind and acts as he preaches? If so, you are a restorative to ailing humanity and a balm for the wounded heart.

The Voice of the Master

KNOWLEDGE IS a light, enriching
The warmth of life, and all may
Partake who seek it out.

The Secrets of the Heart

LEARNING IS the only wealth tyrants cannot despoil. Only death can dim the lamp of knowledge that is within you. The true wealth of a nation lies not in its gold or silver but in its learning, wisdom, and in the uprightness of its sons.

The Voice of the Master

IN EDUCATION the life of the mind proceeds gradually from scientific experiments to intellectual theories, to spiritual feeling, and then to God.

Spiritual Sayings

ON TALKING

YOU BELIEVE in what you hear said. Believe in the unsaid, for the silence of men is nearer the truth than their words.

Jesus, the Son of Man

I COULD NOT talk; so I resorted to silence, the only language of the heart.

The Broken Wings

I SPEAK, my unheeding brothers,
I do indeed speak,
But you hear only your own words.

The Earth Gods

THE TRIBUNE of humanity is in its silent heart, never its talkative mind.

Sand and Foam

SAY OF me what you will and the morrow will judge you, and your words shall be a witness before its judging and a testimony before its justice.

A Tear and a Smile

THE REALITY of the other person is not in what he reveals to you, but in what he cannot reveal to you.
Therefore, if you would understand him, listen not to what he says but rather to what he does not say.

Sand and Foam

WE WERE both silent, each waiting for the other to speak, but speech is not the only means of understanding between two souls. It is not the syllables that come from the lips and tongues that bring hearts together.

There is something greater and purer than what the mouth utters. Silence illuminates our souls, whispers to our hearts, and brings them together. Silence separates us from ourselves, makes us sail the firmament of spirit, and brings us closer to Heaven; it makes us feel that bodies are no more than prisons and that this world is only a place of exile.

The Broken Wings

THE MOST talkative is the least intelligent, and there is hardly a difference between an orator and an auctioneer.

Sand and Foam

I PURIFIED my lips with the sacred fire to speak of love,
But when I opened my lips I found myself speechless.
Before I knew love, I was wont to chant the songs of
    love,
But when I learned to know, the words in my mouth
    became naught save breath,
And the tunes within my breast fell into deep silence.

Prose Poems

YOU SHALL rise beyond your words, but your path shall remain, a rhythm and a fragrance; a rhythm for lovers and for all who are beloved, and a fragrance for those who would live life in a garden.

The Garden of the Prophet

TELL A lovely truth in little words, but never an ugly truth in any words.

The Garden of the Prophet

HALF OF what I say is meaningless; but I say it so that the other half may reach you.

Sand and Foam

HE WHO conceals his intention behind flowery words of praise is like a woman who seeks to hide her ugliness behind cosmetics.

Spiritual Sayings

WORDS ARE timeless. You should utter them or write them with a knowledge of their timelessness.

Sand and Foam

THE ONE who disagrees is more talked about than the one who agrees.

Spiritual Sayings

ONLY THE dumb envy the talkative.

Sand and Foam

THE REAL in us is silent; the acquired is talkative.

Sand and Foam

ON TIME AND PLACE

WE MEASURE time according to the movement of countless suns; and they measure time by little machines in their little pockets.

Now tell me, how could we ever meet at the same place and the same time?

Sand and Foam

HOW STRANGE Time is, and how queer we are! Time has really changed, and lo, it has changed us too. It walked one step forward, unveiled its face, alarmed us and then elated us.

Yesterday we complained about Time and trembled at its terrors. But today we have learned to love it and revere it, for we now understand its intents, its natural disposition, its secrets, and its mysteries.

Thoughts and Meditations

W E OFTEN borrow from our tomorrows to pay our debts to our yesterdays.

Sand and Foam

M Y SOUL preached to me exhorting me not to limit space by saying, 'Here, there, and yonder.' Ere my soul preached to me, I felt that wherever I walked was far from any other space.

Now I realize that wherever I am contains all places; and the distance that I walk embraces all distances.

Thoughts and Meditations

MY SOUL counselled me and admonished me to measure
    time with this saying:
'There was a yesterday and there shall be a tomorrow.'
Unto that hour I deemed the past an epoch that is lost
    and shall be forgotten,
And the future I deemed an era that I may not attain;
But now I have learned this:
That in the brief present all time, with all that is in
    time,
Is achieved and come true.

Prose Poems

WHEN OUT of chaos came the earth, and we, sons of the beginning, beheld each other in the lustless light, we breathed the first hushed, tremulous sound that quickened the currents of air and sea.

Then we walked, hand in hand, upon the grey infant world, and out of the echoes of our first drowsy steps time was born, a fourth divinity, that sets his feet upon our footprints, shadowing our thoughts and desires, and seeing only with our eyes.

The Earth Gods

ON BEAUTY

GREAT BEAUTY captures me, but a beauty still greater frees me even from itself.

Sand and Foam

AFTER A silence, in which were gentle dreams, I asked of her: 'What thing is this beauty? For people differ in its defining and their knowledge thereof as they contend one with another in praise and love of it.'

And she answered: 'It is that which draws your spirit. It is that which you see and makes you to give rather than receive. It is that thing you feel when hands are stretched forth from your depths to clasp it to your depths. It is that which the body reckons a trial and the spirit a bounty. It is the link between joy and sorrow. It is all that you perceive hidden and know unknown and hear silent. It is a Force that begins in the Holy of Holies of your being and ends in that place beyond your visions.'

A Tear and a Smile

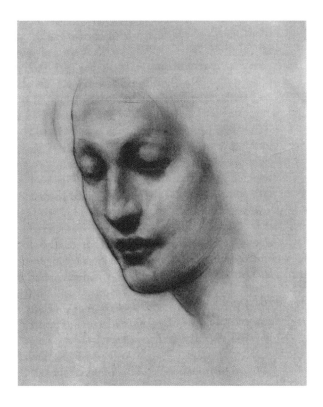

MY SOUL advised me and taught me to perceive the hidden beauty of the skin, figure, and hue. She instructed me to meditate upon that which the people call ugly until its true charm and delight appear.

Thoughts and Meditations

BEAUTY HAS its own heavenly language, loftier than the voices of tongues and lips. It is a timeless language, common to all humanity, a calm lake that attracts the singing rivulets to its depth and makes them silent.

Only our spirits can understand beauty, or live and grow with it. It puzzles our minds; we are unable to describe it in words; it is a sensation that our eyes cannot see, derived from both the one who observes and the one who is looked upon. Real beauty is a ray which emanates from the holy of holies of the spirit, and illuminates the body, as life comes from the depths of the earth and gives colour and scent to a flower.

Real beauty lies in the spiritual accord that is called love which can exist between a man and a woman.

The Broken Wings

I s it not that which you have never striven to reach, into whose heart you have never desired to enter, that you deem ugliness?

The Garden of the Prophet

A re you troubled by the many faiths that Mankind professes? Are you lost in the valley of conflicting beliefs? Do you think that freedom of heresy is less burdensome than the yoke of submission, and the liberty of dissent safer than the stronghold of acquiescence?

If such be the case, then make Beauty your religion, and worship her as your godhead; for she is the visible, manifest and perfect handiwork of God. Cast off those who have toyed with godliness as if it were a sham, joining together greed and arrogance; but believe instead in the divinity of beauty that is at once the beginning of your worship of Life, and the source of your hunger for Happiness.

The Voice of the Master

BEAUTY SHINES brighter in the heart of him who longs for it than in the eyes of him who sees it.

Sand and Foam

THUS, THE appearance of things changes according to the emotions, and thus we see magic and beauty in them, while the magic and beauty are really in ourselves.

The Broken Wings

BEAUTY... IS not the image you would see nor the song you would hear,
But rather an image you see though you close your eyes and a song you hear though you shut your ears.
It is not the sap within the furrowed bark, nor a wing attached to a claw,
But rather a garden for ever in bloom and a flock of angels for ever in flight.

The Prophet

THERE IS neither religion nor science beyond beauty.

Sand and Foam

CALL NOTHING ugly, my friend, save the fear of a soul in the presence of its own memories.

The Garden of Prophet

TO FOLLOW Beauty even when she shall lead you to the verge of the precipice; and though she is wingèd and you are wingless, and though she shall pass beyond the verge, follow her, for where Beauty is not, there is nothing.

The Garden of the Prophet

BEAUTY REVEALS herself to us as she sits on the throne of glory; but we approach her in the name of Lust, snatch off her crown of purity, and pollute her garment with our evil-doing.

The Voice of the Master

LOVE IS forever shy of beauty, yet beauty shall forever be pursued by love.

Jesus, the Son of Man

ON ART

THE ART of the Egyptians is in the occult.
The art of the Chaldeans is in calculation.
The art of the Greeks is in proportion.
The art of the Romans is in echo.
The art of the Chinese is in etiquette.
The art of the Hindus is in the weighing of good
and evil.
The art of the Jews is in the sense of doom.
The art of the Arabs is in reminiscence and
exaggeration.
The art of the Persians is in fastidiousness.
The art of the French is in finesse.
The art of the English is in analysis and self-
righteousness.
The art of the Spaniards is in fanaticism.
The art of the Italians is in beauty.
The art of the Germans is in ambition.
The art of the Russians is in sadness.

Spiritual Sayings

ART BEGAN when man glorified the sun with a hymn of gratitude.

Spiritual Sayings

AND IF there come the singers and the dancers and the flute players – buy of their gifts also.

For they too are gatherers of fruit and frankincense, and that which they bring, though fashioned of dreams, is raiment and food for your soul.

The Prophet

I SHOULD be a traitor to my art if I were to borrow my sitter's eyes. The face is a marvellous mirror that reflects most faithfully the innermost of the soul; the artist's business is to see that and portray it; otherwise he is not fit to be called an artist.

A Biography

ART IS a step from nature toward the Infinite.

Sand and Foam

SOME THINK the business of art to be a mere imitation of nature. But Nature is far too great and too subtle to be successfully imitated. No artist can ever reproduce even the least of Nature's surpassing creations and miracles. Besides, what profit is there in imitating Nature when she is so open and so accessible to all who see and hear? The business of art is rather to understand Nature and to reveal her meanings to those unable to understand. It is to convey the *soul* of a tree rather than to produce a fruitful likeness of the tree. It is to reveal the *conscience* of the sea, not to portray so many foaming waves or so much blue water. The mission of art is to bring out the unfamiliar from the most familiar.

A Biography

ART IS a step in the known toward the unknown.

Spiritual Sayings

I FEEL that art – which is the expression of what floats, moves and becomes an essence in one's *soul* – is more suited and conformable to your rare talents than research – which is the expression of what floats, moves and becomes an essence in *society*.

Love Letters

A WORK of art is a mist carved into an image.

Sand and Foam

I AM [particularly] fond of the antique objects. In the corners of this studio is a small collection of rare and precious things from past ages, such as statues and slates from Egypt, Greece and Rome; Phoenician glass; Persian pottery; ancient books and French and Italian paintings; and musical instruments which speak even in their silence. But some day I must acquire a Chaldean black-stone statue. For I have a special fondness for everything Chaldean; the myths of the Chaldeans, their poetry, their prayers, their geometry, even the minutest relics time has left behind of their art and crafts, all these stir distant and mysterious memories within me, transporting me to days gone by and allowing me to see the past through the window of the future. I love antique objects, and they appeal to me because they are the fruit of human thought marching in a procession of a thousand stamping feet out of the darkness and into the light – that eternal thought which plunges deep down to the bottom of the sea only to rise up to the Milky Way.

Love Letters

ON WISDOM

WISDOM CEASES to be wisdom when it becomes too proud to weep, too grave to laugh, and too self-full to see other than itself.

Sand and Foam

EVERY EVIL has its remedy, except folly.

The Voice of the Master

YOUTH IS a beautiful dream, but its sweetness is enslaved by the dullness of books and its awakening is a harsh one.

Shall there come a day when wise men are able to unite the dreams of youth and the delights of learning as reproach brings together hearts in conflict?

Nymphs of the Valley

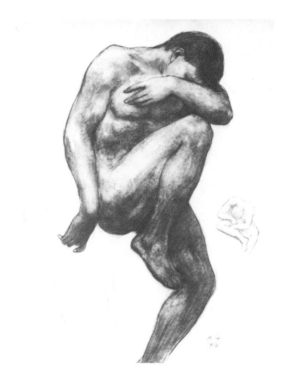

AND I saw Man calling upon Wisdom for deliverance; but Wisdom did not hearken to his cries, for he had contemned her when she spoke to him in the streets of the city.

The Voice of the Master

LEARN THE words of wisdom uttered by the wise and apply them in your own life. Live them – but do not make a show of reciting them, for he who repeats what he does not understand is no better than an ass that is loaded with books.

The Voice of the Master

ON JOY AND SORROW

UPON A day in May, Joy and Sorrow met beside a lake. They greeted one another, and they sat down near the quiet waters and conversed.

Joy spoke of the beauty which is upon the earth, and of the daily wonder of life in the forest and among the hills, and of the songs heard at dawn and eventide.

And Sorrow spoke, and agreed with all that Joy had said; for Sorrow knew the magic of the hour and the beauty thereof. And Sorrow was eloquent when he spoke of May in the fields and among the hills.

And Joy and Sorrow talked long together, and they agreed upon all things of which they knew.

Now there passed by on the other side of the lake two hunters. And as they looked across the water one of them said, 'I wonder who are those two persons?' And the other said, 'Did you say two? I see only one.'

The first hunter said, 'But there are two.' And the second said, 'There is only one that I can see, and the reflection in the lake is only one.'

'Nay, there are two,' said the first hunter, 'and the reflection in the still water is of two persons.'

But the second man said again, 'Only one do I see.' And again the other said, 'But I see two so plainly.'

And even to this day one hunter says that the other sees double; while the other says, 'My friend is somewhat blind.'

The Wanderer

A ND THE God of Gods separated a spirit from Himself and created in it Beauty.

He gave to it the lightness of the breeze at dawn and the fragrance of the flowers of the field and the softness of moonlight.

Then He gave to it a cup of joy, saying,

'You shall not drink of it except that you forget the Past and heed not the Future.'

And He gave to it a cup of sadness, saying,

'You shall drink and know therefrom the meaning of Life's rejoicing.'

A Tear and a Smile

SOME OF you say, 'Joy is greater than sorrow,' and others say, 'Nay, sorrow is the greater.'

But I say unto you, they are inseparable.

Together they come, and when one sits alone with you at your board, remember that the other is asleep upon your bed.

The Prophet

THE SORROWFUL spirit finds rest when united with a similar one...Hearts that are united through the medium of sorrow will not be separated by the glory of happiness. Love that is cleansed by tears will remain eternally pure and beautiful.

The Broken Wings

FOR HE who has not looked on Sorrow will never see Joy.

The Voice of the Master

WHEN EITHER your joy or your sorrow becomes great the world becomes small.

Sand and Foam

You NOW know that sorrow and poverty purify man's heart; though our weak minds see nothing worthy in the universe save ease and happiness.

Thoughts and Meditations

THE BITTEREST thing in our today's sorrow is the memory of our yesterday's joy.

Sand and Foam

FOR WE are all creatures of sadness and of small doubts. And when a man says to us: 'Let us be joyous with the gods,' we cannot but heed his voice.

Jesus, the Son of Man

SORROW SOFTENS the feelings, and Joy heals the wounded heart. Were Sorrow and Poverty abolished, the spirit of man would be like an empty tablet, with naught inscribed save the signs of selfishness and greed.

The Voice of the Master

I WOULD NOT exchange the sorrows of my heart for the joys of the multitude. And I would not have the tears that sadness makes to flow from my every part, turn into laughter. I would that my life remain a tear and a smile.

A Tear and a Smile

WE CHOOSE our joys and our sorrows long before we experience them.

Sand and Foam

YOUR JOY is your sorrow unmasked.

The Prophet

MY SORROWS have taught me to understand the sorrows of my fellow men; neither persecution nor exile have dimmed the vision within me.

The Voice of the Master

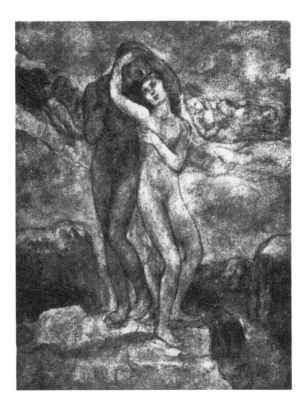

H E WAS a man of joy; and it was upon the path of joy that He met the sorrows of all men.

Jesus, the Son of Man

I F YOU could see, my sorrowful friend, that the misfortune which has defeated you in life is the very power that illumines your heart and raises your soul from the pit of derision to the throne of reverence, you would be content with your share and you would look upon it as a legacy to instruct you and make you wise.

The Voice of the Master

ON FRIENDSHIP

FRIENDSHIP IS always a sweet responsibility, never an opportunity.

Sand and Foam

IF YOU do not understand your friend under all conditions you will never understand him.

Sand and Foam

YOUR FRIEND is your needs answered.
He is your field which you sow with love and reap with
    thanksgiving.
And he is your board and your fireside.
For you come to him with your hunger, and you seek
    him for peace.

The Prophet

MY FRIEND, thou art not my friend, but how shall I make thee understand? My path is not thy path, yet together we walk, hand in hand.

The Madman

AND LET there be no purpose in friendship save the deepening of the spirit.

For love that seeks aught but the disclosure of its own mystery is not love but a net cast forth: and only the unprofitable is caught.

The Prophet

FRIENDSHIP WITH the ignorant is as foolish as arguing with a drunkard.

The Voice of the Master

ON EATING AND DRINKING

THE TREE of my heart is heavy with fruit. Come, ye hungry souls, gather it, eat and be satisfied. My spirit overflows with aged wine. Come, oh ye thirsty hearts, drink and quench your thirst.

The Voice of the Master

ONCE A man sat at my board and ate my bread and drank my wine and went away laughing at me.
Then he came again for bread and wine, and I spurned him;
And the angels laughed at me.

Sand and Foam

YOU DRINK wine that you may be intoxicated; and I drink that it may sober me from that other wine.

Sand and Foam

ONCE THERE lived a rich man who was justly proud of his cellar and the wine therein. And there was one jug of ancient vintage kept for some occasion known only to himself.

The governor of the state visited him, and he bethought him and said, 'That jug shall not be opened for a mere governor.'

And a bishop of the diocese visited him, but he said to himself, 'Nay, I will not open that jug. He would not know its value, nor would its aroma reach his nostrils.'

The prince of the realm came and supped with him. But he thought, 'It is too royal a wine for a mere princeling.'

And even on the day when his own nephew was married, he said to himself, 'No, not to these guests shall that jug be brought forth.'

And the years passed by, and he died, an old man, and he was buried like unto every seed and acorn.

And upon the day that he was buried the ancient jug was brought out together with other jugs of wine, and it was shared by the peasants of the neighbourhood. And none knew its great age.

To them, all that is poured into a cup is only wine.

The Wanderer

AND IN the autumn, when you gather the grapes of your vineyards for the winepress, say in your heart,
'I too am a vineyard, and my fruit shall be gathered for the winepress,
And like new wine I shall be kept in eternal vessels.'
And in winter, when you draw the wine, let there be in your heart a song for each cup;
And let there be in the song a remembrance for the autumn days, and for the vineyard, and for the winepress.

The Prophet

WHEN MY cup is empty I resign myself to its emptiness; but when it is half full I resent its half-fullness.

Sand and Foam

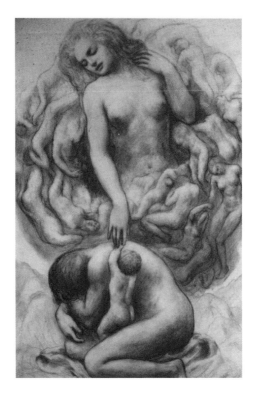

ON HOUSES

BUILD OF your imaginings a bower in the wilderness ere you build a house within the city walls.

The Prophet

AND TELL me, people of Orphalese, what have you in these houses? And what is it you guard with fastened doors?

Have you peace, the quiet urge that reveals your power?

Have you remembrances, the glimmering arches that span the summits of the mind?

Have you beauty, that leads the heart from things fashioned of wood and stone to the holy mountain?

Tell me, have you these in your houses?

Or have you only comfort, and the lust for comfort, that stealthy thing that enters the house a guest, and then becomes a host, and then a master?

The Prophet

I N THEIR fear your forefathers gathered you too near together. And that fear shall endure a little longer. A little longer shall your city walls separate your hearths from your fields.

The Prophet

B UT YOU, children of space, you restless in rest, you shall not be trapped nor tamed.

Your house shall be not an anchor but a mast.

It shall not be a glistening film that covers a wound, but an eyelid that guards the eye.

You shall not fold your wings that you may pass through doors, nor bend your heads that they strike not against a ceiling, nor fear to breathe lest walls should crack and fall down.

You shall not dwell in tombs made by the dead for the living.

And though of magnificence and splendour, your house shall not hold your secret nor shelter your longing.

For that which is boundless in you abides in the mansion of the sky, whose door is the morning mist, and whose windows are the songs and the silences of night.

The Prophet

DOES NOT your house dream? and dreaming, leave the city for grove or hill-top?

The Prophet

IF IT were not for guests, all houses would be graves.

Sand and Foam

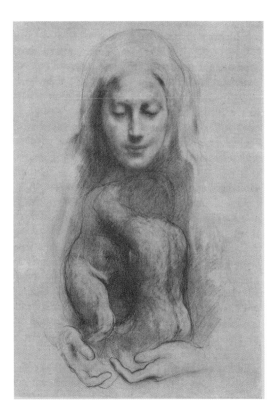

ON BUYING AND SELLING

AND BEFORE you leave the market place, see that no one
    has gone his way with empty hands.
For the master spirit of the earth shall not sleep peace-
    fully upon the wind till the needs of the least of you
    are satisfied.

The Prophet

ARE YOU a merchant, drawing advantage from the needs of
the people, engrossing goods so as to resell them at an
exorbitant price? If so, you are a reprobate; and it
matters naught whether your home is a palace or a prison.

Or are you an honest man, who enables farmer and weaver to
exchange their products, who mediates between buyer and
seller, and through his just ways profits both himself and
others?

If so, you are a righteous man; and it matters not whether
you are praised or blamed.

The Voice of the Master

WHAT SHALL I say about him who borrows from me the money to buy a sword with which to attack me?

Spiritual Sayings

THEY DEEM me mad because I will not sell my days for gold;
And I deem them mad because they think my days have a price.

Sand and Foam

IF YOUR knowledge teaches you not the value of things, and frees you not from the bondage to matter, you shall never come near the throne of Truth.

The Voice of the Master

THE MOST pitiful among men is he who turns his dreams into silver and gold.

Sand and Foam

WHEN IN the market place you toilers of the sea and
   fields and vineyards meet the weavers and the
   potters and the gatherers of spices–
Invoke then the master spirit of the earth, to come into
   your midst and sanctify the scales and the reckoning
   that weighs value against value.

And suffer not the barren-handed to take part in your
   transactions, who would sell their words for your
   labour.
To such men you should say,
'Come with us to the field, or go with our brothers to the
   sea and cast your net;
For the land and the sea shall be bountiful to you even
   as to us.'

The Prophet

ON OTHER MATTERS

SEEMING IS but a garment I wear – a care-woven garment that protects me from thy questionings and thee from my negligence.

The Madman

PRAYER IS the song of the heart that makes its way to the throne of God even when entangled in the wailing of thousands of souls.

Spiritual Sayings

YOU PRAY in your distress and in your need; would that you might pray also in the fullness of your joy and in your days of abundance.

The Prophet

REMEMBER, ONE just man causes the Devil greater affliction than a million blind believers.

The Voice of the Master

YOU ARE my brother and I love you, and love is justice in its highest manifestation.

A Tear and a Smile

THEN I knew at once the meaning of the Wardé's story and understood the secret of her protest against a society that persecutes the rebel against its edicts before knowing the cause of his rebellion.

Spirits Rebellious

DO NOT expect good counsel from a tyrant, or a wrong-doer, or a presumptuous man, or a deserter from honour. Woe to him who conspires with the wrongdoer who comes seeking advice. For to agree with the wrongdoer is infamy, and to hearken to that which is false is treachery.

The Voice of the Master

WHERE IS the justice of sovereignty when it slays the slayer and imprisons the robber and then falls upon its neighbour and kills and plunders in its thousands?

A Tear and a Smile

U PON A day Beauty and Ugliness met on the shore of a sea. And they said to one another, 'Let us bathe in the sea.'

Then they disrobed and swam in the waters. And after a while Ugliness came back to shore and garmented himself with the garments of Beauty and walked his way.

And Beauty too came out of the sea, and found not her raiment, and she was too shy to be naked, therefore she dressed herself with the raiment of Ugliness. And Beauty walked her way.

And to this very day men and women mistake the one for the other.

Yet some there are who have beheld the face of Beauty, and they know her notwithstanding her garments. And some there be who know the face of Ugliness, and the cloth conceals him not from their eyes.

The Wanderer

L ET HIM who wipes his soiled hands with your garment take your garment. He may need it again; surely you would not.

Sand and Foam

YOUR CLOTHES conceal much of your beauty, yet they hide not the unbeautiful.

And though you seek in garments the freedom of privacy you may find in them a harness and a chain.

Would that you could meet the sun and the wind with more of your skin and less of your raiment,

For the breath of life is in the sunlight and the hand of life is in the wind.

The Prophet

THE OTHER day I saw a rich man standing at the temple door, stretching out his hands, which were full of precious stones, toward all passers-by, and calling to them, saying: 'Have pity on me. Take these jewels from me. For they have made my soul sick and hardened my heart. Pity me, take them, and make me whole again.'

The Voice of the Master

DO NOT the spirits who dwell in the ether envy man his pain?

Sand and Foam

MY FELLOW poor, Poverty sets off the nobility of the spirit, while wealth discloses its evil. Sorrow softens the feelings, and Joy heals the wounded heart. Were Sorrow and Poverty abolished, the spirit of man would be like an empty tablet, with naught inscribed save the signs of selfishness and greed.

The Voice of the Master

YOUR LIFE, my fellow men, is an island separated from all other islands and regions. No matter how many are the ships that leave your shores for other climes, no matter how many are the fleets that touch your coast, you remain a solitary island, suffering the pangs of loneliness and yearning for happiness. You are unknown to your fellow men and far removed from their sympathy and understanding.

The Voice of the Master

THE PHILOSOPHER'S soul dwells in his head, the poet's soul is in his heart; the singer's soul lingers about his throat, but the soul of the dancer abides in all her body.

The Wanderer

WE ARE neither able nor willing to touch the sides of the altar save with hands that have been purified by fire. And when we love a thing…we look on love as a goal in itself and not as a means to achieve some other end; and if we show reverence and submission before the sublime, it is because we regard submission as elevation and reverence as a form of recompense. If we long for something, we consider longing a gift and a bounty in itself. We also know that the remotest matters are those most befitting and most worthy of our longing and our inclinations. In truth we two – you and I – cannot stand in the light of the sun and say: 'We must spare ourselves torment we can well do without.' We cannot do without that which infuses the soul with a sacred leaven, nor can we do without the caravan which takes us to God's city; indeed we cannot do without that which brings us nearer to our Greater Selves and reveals to us the power, mystery and wonder we have within our souls. Moreover we are capable of finding intellectual happiness in the simplest manifestations of the soul for in a simple flower we find all the glory and beauty of spring, in the eyes of the infant suckling we find all the hope and aspiration of mankind.

Love Letters

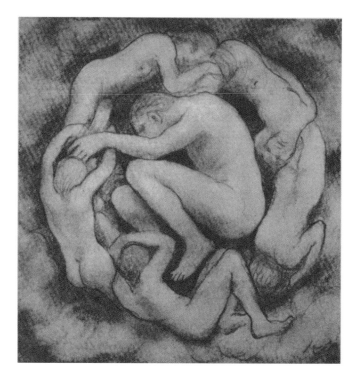

FOR WE could not hear the song of the bodiless wind nor see our greater self walking in the mist.

Jesus, the Son of Man

YOUR NEIGHBOUR is your other self dwelling behind a wall. In understanding, all walls shall fall down.

Jesus, the Son of Man

YOU ARE but a fragment of your giant self, a mouth that seeks bread, and a blind hand that holds the cup for a thirsty mouth.

Sand and Foam

MY FRIEND, be not like him who sits by his fireside and watches the fire go out, then blows vainly upon the dead ashes. Do not give up hope or yield to despair because of that which is past, for to bewail the irretrievable is the worst of human frailties.

The Voice of the Master

PITY THE nation that wears a cloth it does not weave, eats a bread it does not harvest, and drinks a wine that flows not from its own winepress.

Pity the nation that acclaims the bully as hero, and that deems the glittering conqueror bountiful.

Pity a nation that despises a passion in its dream, yet submits in its awakening.

Pity the nation that raises not its voice save when it walks in a funeral, boasts not except among its ruins, and will rebel not save when its neck is laid between the sword and the block.

Pity the nation whose statesman is a fox, whose philosopher is a juggler, and whose art is the art of patching and mimicking.

Pity the nation that welcomes its new ruler with trumpetings, and farewells him with hootings, only to welcome another with trumpetings again.

Pity the nation whose sages are dumb with years and whose strong men are yet in the cradle.

Pity the nation divided into fragments, each fragment deeming itself a nation.

The Garden of the Prophet

H E DID not utterly condemn the liar or the thief or the murderer, but He did utterly condemn the hypocrite whose face is masked and whose hand is gloved.

Jesus, the Son of Man

W EAKLINGS, WHOM you call sinners, are like the featherless young that fall from the nest. The hypocrite is the vulture waiting upon a rock for the death of the prey.

Jesus, the Son of Man

B ABYLON WAS not put to waste by her prostitutes; Babylon fell to ashes that the eyes of her hypocrites might no longer see the light of day.

Jesus, the Son of Man

A BLESSING

BLESSED ARE the serene in spirit.

Blessed are they who are not held by possessions, for they shall be free.

Blessed are they who remember their pain, and in their pain await their joy.

Blessed are they who hunger after truth and beauty, for their hunger shall bring bread, and their thirst cool water.

Blessed are the kindly, for they shall be consoled by their own kindliness.

Blessed are the pure in heart, for they shall be one with God.

Blessed are the merciful, for mercy shall be in their portion.

Blessed are the peacemakers, for their spirit shall dwell above the battle, and they shall turn the potter's field into a garden.

Blessed are they who are hunted, for they shall be swift of foot and they shall be wingèd.

Jesus, the Son of Man

A CHRONOLOGY OF THE
LIFE OF KAHLIL GIBRAN

1883   Gibran Khalil Gibran[1] was born on January 6 near the Holy Cedar Grove on the edge of Wadi Qadisha (The Holy or Sacred Valley) in the town of Bisharri, Lebanon. His mother Kamileh, the daughter of a clergyman, named Istiphan Rahmeh, was a widow when she married Khalil Gibran, father of the poet. Kamileh's first husband was Hanna Abd-es-Salaam Rahmeh, by whom she had one son, Boutros, who was six years old when Gibran was born.

1885   Miriana, Gibran's first sister, was born.

---

[1] Gibran's full name in Arabic was Gibran Khalil Gibran, the middle name being his father's. It is a convention among the Arabs to use the father's name after one's first name. He always signed his full name in his Arabic works, but dropped the first name in his English writings. He did this, and changed the correct spelling of 'Khalil' into 'Kahlil', at the instigation of his teacher of English at the Boston school he attended between 1895 and 1897.

1887   Sultanah, Gibran's second sister, was born.

1895   Kahlil, his half-brother Boutros, his mother, and his two sisters emigrated to the United States, settling in Boston's Chinatown, while his father remained in Lebanon.

1897   Gibran returned to Lebanon, where he began a course of intensive study at al-Hikmah School. He studied a wide variety of subjects beyond those prescribed in the curriculum, and immersed himself in Arabic literature, ancient and modern. He also familiarized himself with contemporary literary movements in the Arab world.

1899   During the summer vacation at Bisharri, Gibran fell desperately in love with a beautiful young woman. Although there is much conjecture as to the nature of this relationship and the identity of the young woman, it is certain that Gibran found his first love-affair both frustrating and disappointing. In the autumn he returned to Boston by way of Paris, and several years later described the unhappy affair in *The Broken Wings*.

1902   Gibran returned to Lebanon once more, this time as a guide and interpreter to an American family, but was forced to hurry back to Boston on hearing of the death of his sister, Sultanah, and of the serious illness of his mother.

1903   In March his half-brother Boutros died, and his mother died in June, leaving Gibran and his sister Miriana in Boston. His mother, half-brother, and younger sister all died of tuberculosis.

1904   By now Gibran was beginning to attract attention as an artist. Fred Holland Day, a well-known photographer, became Gibran's first patron, holding at his studio in January an exhibition of the poet's paintings and drawings. In February a second exhibition was held at the Cambridge School, a private educational institution owned and operated by Mary Haskell, who became Gibran's close friend, patroness and benefactress.

At the Cambridge School he also met a beautiful and impulsive young woman of French origin, Emilie Michel, who was known to all her acquaintances as Micheline and with whom, it is said, Gibran fell in love.

1905   Gibran published *al-Musiqah (Music)*, his first book in Arabic.

1906   Gibran published a savage attack against the Church and the State in *'Ara'is al-Muruj (Nymphs of the Valley)*, which earned him the reputation of being a rebel and a revolutionary, a reputation which the publication of his later mystical works only partially mitigated.

1908   Besides arranging for the publication of *al-Arwah al-Mutamarridah (Spirits Rebellious)*, Gibran also worked on *Falsafat al-Din wa'l-Tadayyun (The Philosophy of Religion and Religiosity)*, which was never published.

      Through the generosity of Mary Haskell, who was determined to help Gibran fulfil his ambition to become a great artist and thinker, he went to Paris, visiting London on the way, to study art at the Académie Julien and at the Ecoles des Beaux-Arts.

      During his stay in Paris he came into contact with European literature, and read the works of contemporary English and French writers. He also became especially interested in the work of William Blake, who greatly influenced his thought and art; and for a while fell under the spell of Friedrich Nietzsche's *Thus Spake Zarathustra*; but Nietzsche's influence, unlike that of Blake, was short-lived.

1909   Gibran continued his studies in Paris, where he met again an old classmate from al-Hikmah, Yusuf al-Huwayik, also an art student. The two men became close friends, and together tried to acquaint themselves with modern trends in painting. They found, however, that they had little sympathy with Cubism, which one of them described as a 'lunatic revolution', and instead reaffirmed their loyalty to the classical tradition. They also met the sculptor Auguste Rodin, and although this meeting lasted only for a few seconds, Rodin was to exert a powerful influence on Gibran's art. His teacher in Paris was in fact Maître Lawrence, whose art Gibran so detested that eventually he left him and began to work on his own.

Gibran's father died in Lebanon.

1910   Gibran, Ameen Rihani, and Yusuf al-Huwayik met in London and laid many plans for a cultural renaissance of the Arab world. Among these plans was one for the founding of an opera house in Beirut, the outstanding feature of which was to be two domes symbolising the reconciliation between Christianity and Islam.

After his return to Boston in October, Gibran proposed marriage to Mary Haskell, who was ten years his senior, but he was not accepted.

1911   At a time of intense political activity occasioned by the freeing of Arab territories from Ottoman rule, Gibran founded *'al-Halqa' l-Dhahabiyyah* (*The Golden Circle*), one of many semi-political Arab societies which sprang up in Syria, Lebanon, Constantinople, Paris and New York. But the Golden Circle was not popular among Arab immigrants and was dissolved after the first meeting.

Gibran began to earn his living through portrait painting.

1912   Gibran moved from Boston to New York, where he hired a studio at 51 West Tenth Street, between Fifth and Sixth Avenue. 'The Hermitage', as Gibran called his studio, remained his home until his death. He published *al-Ajnihah 'l-Mutakassirah* (*The Broken*

Wings), his autobiographical narrative, on which he had been working since 1903.

In April he met 'Abdu'l-Bahá and made a drawing of him. This meeting left an indelible impression on Gibran's thought which lasted to the end of his life.

A literary and love relationship began between Gibran and May Ziadah, a Lebanese writer living in Egypt. Although they knew each other only through their correspondence, which lasted for more than twenty years, they achieved a rare intimacy and harmony of understanding which was broken only by Gibran's death.

1914   Gibran collected a number of his prose poems which had appeared in different magazines since 1904, and published them under the title *Dam'ah wa'Ibtisamah (A Tear and a Smile)*. In December an exhibition of his paintings and drawings was held at the Montross Galleries, New York.

1917   Two other exhibitions of Gibran's works were held: one at the Knoedler Galleries, New York; the other at the Doll and Richards Galleries, Boston.

1918   Gibran published *The Madman*, his first book written in English.

1919   Gibran published *Twenty Drawings*, a collection of his drawings with an introduction by Alice Raphael, and also *al-Mawakib (The Procession)*, a philosophical poem illustrated by Gibran himself and containing some of his best drawings.

1920   In addition to publishing *al-'Awasif (The Tempests)*, a collection of short narratives and prose poems which had appeared in various journals between 1912 and 1918, and his second English book, *The Forerunner*, Gibran became founder-president of a literary society called *al-Rabita 'l-Qalamiyyah (Arrabitah)*, which exerted a powerful influence on the work of immigrant Arab poets (Shu'ara' 'l-Mahjar) and on successive generations of Arab writers.

1921   Gibran published a thematic 'play', *Iram Dhat al-Imad (Iram, City of Lofty Pillars)*, written in Arabic and taking the form of a discourse on mysticism.

His health began to deteriorate.

1922   In January another exhibition of his work was held in Boston, this time at the Women's City Club.

1923   Gibran published *al-Badayi'wa'l-Tarayif (Beautiful and Rare Sayings)* in which he included his own sketches (drawn from imagination when he was seventeen) of some of the greatest Arab philosophers and poets such as Ibn Sina (Avicenna), Al Ghazzali, al-Khansa', Ibn al-Farid, Abu Nuwas, Ibn al-Muqafa' and others.

       He published *The Prophet*, his most successful work.

1926   Gibran published *Sand and Foam*, a book of aphorisms some of which were first written in Arabic and then translated into English.

1928   Gibran published *Jesus, The Son of Man*, his longest work.

1931   Two weeks before his death, he published *The Earth Gods*. Gibran died on Friday, April 10, at St. Vincent's Hospital, New York, after a long and painful illness, described in the autopsy as 'cirrhosis of the liver with incipient tuberculosis in one of the lungs'. His body lay in a funeral parlour for two days and thousands of admirers came to pay their last respects. It was then taken to Boston, where a funeral service was conducted in the Church of our Lady of the Cedars. The body was then taken to a vault to await its return to Lebanon, where it arrived at the port of Beirut on August 21. After a magnificent reception unique in the history of Lebanon, Gibran's body was carried to Bisharri to its final resting place in the old chapel of the Monastery of Mar Sarkis. Not far from Mar Sarkis a permanent Gibran museum has been established by the people of Bisharri with the sponsorship and encouragement of the Government of Lebanon. At his death, Gibran left two works which were published posthumously: the completed *Wanderer*, which appeared in 1932; and the unfinished *Garden of the Prophet*, which was completed and published in 1933 by Barbara Young, an American poetess who claimed to have been Gibran's companion during the last seven years of his life.

BIBLIOGRAPHY

The following are the sources from which all the quotations in this anthology have been extracted.

Beloved Prophet: The Love Letters of Kahlil Gibran and Mary Haskell and her Private Journal. Edited and arranged by Virginia Hilu. New York: Alfred A. Knopf, 1972.

Between Night and Morn: A Special Selection. Translated by A. R. Ferris. New York: The Wisdom Library, 1972.

The Broken Wings. Translated by A. R. Ferris. London: Heinemann, 1959. Reprinted, 1961.

The Earth Gods. London: Heinemann, 1962. Reprinted, 1971.

The Forerunner: His Parables and Poems. London: Heinemann, 1963. Reprinted, 1972.

The Garden of the Prophet. London: Heinemann, 1934. Reprinted, 1961.

Jesus, the Son of Man: His Words and his Deeds as Told and Recorded by Those who Knew Him. London: Heinemann, 1928. Reprinted, 1969.

Kahlil Gibran: A Biography, by Mikhail Naimy. New York: Philosophical Library, 1950. Reprinted, 1985.

Kahlil Gibran: A Self-Portrait. Translated and edited by A. R. Ferris. New York: The Citadel Press, 1969.

The Life of Kahlil Gibran and his Procession. Edited, translated, and with a biographical sketch by G. Kheirallah. New York: The Wisdom Library, 1958.

Love Letters. Translated and edited by S. B. Bushrui and S. H. al-Kuzbari. Oxford: Oneworld, 1999.

The Madman: His Parables and Poems. London: Heinemann, 1963. Reprinted, 1971.

Mirrors of the Soul. Translated with biographical notes by J. Sheban. NewYork: Philosophical Library, 1965.

Nymphs of the Valley. Translated by H. M. Nahmad. London: Heinemann, 1948. Reprinted, 1961.

The Prophet. New York: Alfred A. Knopf, 1923. Reprint, 1998.

Prose Poems. Translated by A. Ghareeb. London: Heinemann, 1964. Reprinted, 1972.

Sand and Foam. London: Heinemann, 1927. Reprinted, 1954.

The Secrets of the Heart: A Special Selection. Translated by A. R. Ferris and edited by M. L. Wolf. New York: The Wisdom Library, 1971.

Spirits Rebellious. Translated by H. M. Nahmad. New York: Alfred A. Knopf, 1948. Reprinted, 1963.

Spiritual Sayings. Translated and edited by A. R. Ferris. London: Heinemann, 1963. Reprinted, 1974.

A Tear and a Smile. Translated by H. M. Nahmad. London: Heinemann, 1950. Reprinted, 1972.

Thoughts and Meditations. Translated and edited by A. R. Ferris. New York: The Citadel Press, 1969.

A Treasury of Kahlil Gibran. Translated by A. R. Ferris and edited by M. L. Wolf. New York: The Citadel Press, 1965.

The Voice of the Master. Translated by A. R. Ferris. London: Heinemann, 1960. Reprinted, 1973.

The Wanderer: His Parables and his Sayings. London: Heinemann, 1965. Reprinted, 1972.

ACKNOWLEDGEMENTS

In the preparation of this volume I have received much valuable help from Miss Sepedeh Hooshidari, Miss Poupak Moallem, Mr Mike Dravis, Mr Siamak Majidi and Mr Nabil Bashirelahi.

Acknowledgement is extended to The Citadel Press for extracts from *The Broken Wings, Kahlil Gibran: A Self Portrait, Secrets of the Heart, A Treasury of Kahlil Gibran, The Voice of the Master* • William Heinemann Ltd. for extracts from *The Voice of the Master* • Mrs G. Kheirallah for extracts from *The Procession* • Mr Mikhail Naimy for extracts from *Kahlil Gibran: A Biography* • Philosophical Library, Inc. for extracts from *Between Night and Morn:* copyright 1972, and *Mirrors of the Soul:* copyright 1965 • Anthony R. Ferris for extracts from *Spiritual Sayings*: copyright 1962, and *Thoughts and Meditations*: copyright 1960 • *Love Letters* © S.B. Bushrui and Salma Haffar al-Kusbari 1983, 1995, 1999 •